the
natural woman

the natural woman

gentle healing
and beauty
wisdom for
women of
every age

Shirley Price • Janet Wright • Jennifer Amerena
Photography by Michelle Garrett and Liz McAulay

LORENZ BOOKS

This edition is published by Lorenz Books

Lorenz Books is an imprint of Anness Publishing Ltd
Hermes House, 88-89 Blackfriars Road, London SE1 8HA
tel. 020 7401 2077; fax 020 7633 9499
www.lorenzbooks.com; info@anness.com

© Anness Publishing Ltd 2003

This edition distributed in the UK by Aurum Press Ltd,
25 Bedford Avenue, London WC1B 3AT
tel. 020 7637 3225; fax 020 7580 2469

This edition distributed in the USA and Canada by
National Book Network, 4720 Boston Way, Lanham, MD 20706
tel. 301 459 3366; fax 301 459 1705; www.nbnbooks.com

This edition distributed in Australia by Pan Macmillan Australia,
Level 18, St Martins Tower, 31 Market St, Sydney, NSW 2000
tel. 1300 135 113; fax 1300 135 103
customer.service@macmillan.com.au

This edition distributed in New Zealand by David Bateman Ltd,
30 Tarndale Grove, Off Bush Road, Albany, Auckland
tel. (09) 415 7664; fax (09) 415 8892

Publisher: Joanna Lorenz
Managing Editor: Helen Sudell
Editors: Sarah Ainsley, Melanie Halton, Ann Kay
Herbal Text on p248-251: Jessica Houdret
Designer: Lisa Tai, Ann Cannings, Andrew Nash
Photographers: Liz McAuley, Michelle Garrett
Editorial Reader: Jay Thundercliffe
Production Controller: Wendy Lawson

Previously published in three separate volumes, *Aromatherapy for Women*,
Ayurvedic Beauty and *Aging Naturally*

10 9 8 7 6 5 4 3 2 1

Contents

introduction

Since time began human beings have sought to improve their health and well-being through ingenious use of the materials around them. Natural medicines were probably the first discoveries in this field, but it wasn't long before people looked for ways of doing more than just survive. They used the natural healing properties of herbs and flowers as preventative treatments too.

Our ancestors were using herbal powders and creams thousands of years ago — we know because they were buried with these valuable items beside them for use in the afterlife. They may have started out using an oil to help an injury heal, then discovered that it left their skin feeling more supple or protected it from the weather. If the sheen highlighted their cheekbones, all the better. Health, beauty and well-being were beginning to be developed hand in hand.

Over the centuries we've discovered ever more sophisticated ways of improving our health, enhancing our looks and staying youthful. The range of products now at our disposal would bewilder even our grandmothers. We can conquer infections or delay the

▽ Choosing delicious, fresh fruit as an alternative to stodgy snacks is a simple way of beginning a healthier way of life.

menopause with drugs they had never heard of, and undergo surgery to wipe the marks of time off our faces.

But if the 20th century offered us quick fixes in abundance, it also taught us that there's a price to pay in the form of side effects, allergies and environmental damage. Our understanding of the natural world has been outstripped by our ability to manipulate it.

In the 21st century we are learning to evaluate new products and technologies more realistically. We don't want to hand our children a polluted, depleted world full of drug-resistant diseases. We are rediscovering the wisdom of our ancestors and learning to value what other cultures have to offer. Today, we can pick and mix from a treasure-trove of options: modern, traditional and worldwide.

This beautiful book is for anyone who wants to make the most of every stage of her life. "Natural" doesn't mean refusing the benefits of the world we were born into. We're happy to use medicinal drugs, for example, as long as they work without causing harm. If we don't need them, we'd rather try gentle remedies such as essential oils or Ayurvedic massage.

Medical science now proves that a healthy lifestyle can slow down the aging process and improve our looks and vitality at any age. The three sections of this book approach this from different directions, together building a resource for use throughout life.

The rapidly growing popularity of complementary therapies has brought aromatherapy into the mainstream. But, as world-renowned pioneer Shirley Price explains, the reality is much less widely understood. Far from simply inspiring a range of nice-smelling toiletries, this therapy can relieve many ailments, both physical and psychological. A drop of lavender oil on a pillow has for generations offered gentler relief from insomnia than anything a doctor could prescribe. But who would have thought of blending it in a compress with basil and sweet marjoram to relieve period pains? Or dripping it onto a teabag to ease post-menopausal aching joints?

This section is also packed with easy-to-make recipes for creams and scrubs, widely used in India but rarely written down. These authentic recipes were contributed by beauty therapist Yasmin Sadikot and other women who have adapted their traditional Indian family lore to suit a modern lifestyle.

One great change from our ancestors' time is in our lifespans. Surviving longer than ever before, women in developed countries can now expect to live for nearly 30 years after the menopause. Time to relax and enjoy all the pleasures of a more leisurely life — as long as you stay healthy and able-bodied.

In Aging Naturally there is ample self-help information that can make this a long and rewarding period of any woman's life. Almonds and pumpkin seeds, for example, provide vital minerals to keep bones healthy. Adding a few flexibility exercises to your daily routine can release a grace of movement you never thought possible. So don't wait till you start slowing down before making some life-enhancing changes — now's the time to start getting more out of life, the natural way.

▽ Fresh flowers bring beauty into our lives and stimulate feelings of happiness and well-being.

△ Many different plant extracts are used in beauty products. An extract is chosen not only for its fragrance, but also for its healing properties.

Healing Aromatherapy offers ideas for health and well-being at all stages of a woman's life. It describes what aromatic essential oils are, how they work and which oils and blends can be used to target specific problems and restore the mind–body harmony that is needed for good health.

In Ayurvedic Beauty, the ancient Indian system that covers all aspects of human life is explored. Ayurveda's rules for healthy living, laid down 3,000 years ago, are still relevant today. Beauty shines through skin nourished by pure food, from a mind and body that work harmoniously — with stress relieved by meditation and a body tuned by yoga. It is enhanced by treatments refined during centuries of safe and effective use.

Healing
Aromatherapy

What is aromatherapy?

Many books have been written on the subject of aromatherapy. This section aims to be a little different in that it will illustrate how any woman can benefit from using essential oils throughout the stages of her life – beginning with the onset of puberty, through pregnancy and her reproductive years, on to the menopause and beyond. The section gives profiles of some of the most commonly used oils and describes how they can be used to treat physical and emotional conditions and to alleviate stress. It gives an overview of essential oils and offers advice for the best methods of use in the home. It also describes how oils can be incorporated into a woman's daily skin and beauty regime. First though, it is important to understand what is meant by aromatherapy, as well as something of how it works.

A popular conception of aromatherapy is as a "massage using essential oils". Although there is a connection between massage and aromatherapy, it is not strictly correct to define one in terms of the other.

Aromatherapy has been defined as "the controlled and knowledgeable use of essential oils for therapeutic purposes". These oils are powerful substances and they should always be handled with care, with professional advice taken where necessary. The essential oils used in aromatherapy are not the same as those used by the perfume and food industries, which standardize or adulterate them for commercial interest. Essential oils for aromatherapy should be natural, with nothing added or taken away.

◁ Many different plant extracts are used in beauty products. An extract is chosen not only for its fragrance, but also for its healing properties.

▷ Essential oils can be applied on a compress. Cut up pieces of cotton material and soak them in an oil and water preparation.

▷ Vaporizing special aromatherapy candles is an easy way to set the mood for any occasion.

△ Adding a few drops of essential oil to a saucer of water and heating it over a candle flame causes the oil to vaporize and release its aroma into the room.

How to use this section

When essential oils are used for pleasure alone, the choice of oil is usually based on an individual's preferred aroma, and the properties and effects of the oil are not a priority. However, when used to maintain or improve health, the properties and effects are an important part of the choice.

Each essential oil has many properties, and these can affect both body and mind in more than one way. For example, rosemary essential oil has analgesic properties which will benefit headaches, painful digestion and muscular pain. However, rosemary is also a neurotonic, and can relieve general fatigue and stimulate the memory.

At the end of each chapter of this section is a list of essential oils recommended to help problems associated with that stage in life. Next to each one, from the oil's many assets, are shown the properties relevant to

the particular problem. As an example, where geranium is suggested for athlete's foot, its antifungal quality is listed because this is the property required. In another case, where geranium is suggested for diarrhoea, its anti-inflammatory, antispasmodic and astringent properties are given because these are the relevant properties.

An enhanced result can often be obtained by selecting and using more than one essential oil (two, three or even four different essential oils can be used to make up the required number of drops). The synergy of the blended oils will result in an increase of energy within the mix, when compared to the energy available from one single essential oil.

Having selected the oils you want to use, the chapter on Aromatherapy Techniques will show you how to prepare them for use.

The application techniques suitable for use at home are shown here – application to the skin in a carrier oil, which takes the oils into the bloodstream and all around the body, or by inhalation alone. When we breathe in, some essential oil molecules travel to the lungs to be absorbed into the blood. Other molecules go directly to the brain. This is the quickest route and the most effective way to heal weak or fragile emotions and states of mind, such as stress and depression. The nose not only warms and cleans the inhaled air, but it also enables us to identify substances by their smell. Tiny hairs in the human nose, called cilia, send information via receptor cells to the brain to identify the inhaled molecules. The brain then releases neurochemicals, and these have either a sedative or a tonic effect, depending on the aroma.

The essential oils

Essential oils are powerful agents and all of them – even those nominated as safe – must be used in the correct amounts and for the conditions to which they are best suited. One or two pure essential oils, and most synthetic and adulterated ones, may cause irritation and skin sensitivity. The botanical varieties chosen for this book have been carefully selected from those which do not present this problem. However, these varieties are not always commonly available in the shops and appropriate cautions are included here for the sake of safety.

Except in emergencies, as in cases of burns, stings or wounds, essential oils should not be applied undiluted to the skin, but should be mixed first in a base carrier oil. Citrus oils are photosensitive and should not be used before sunbathing. If you are unsure about the suitability of an oil, always seek the advice of a qualified aromatherapist.

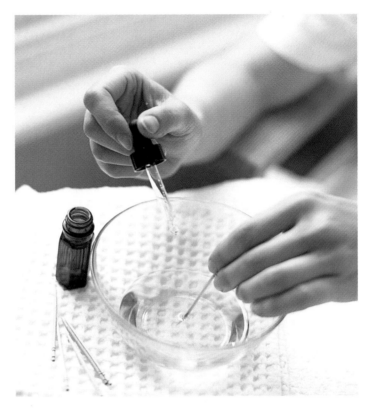

◁ **Prepare a compress for treatment at home by blending your favourite essential oils and adding them to water.**

▽ **Setting the scene at home will contribute to the benefits of aromatherapy. Choose a quiet part of the house and light candles to help you relax.**

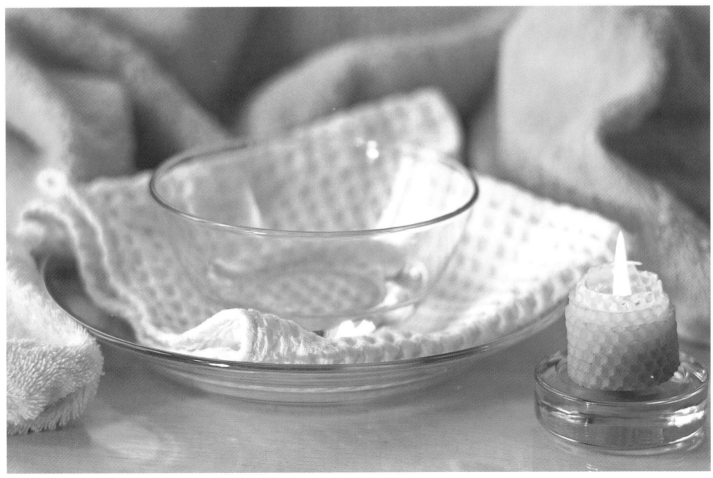

Boswellia carteri – frankincense
family *Burseraceae*

properties
analgesic, anti-infectious, antioxidant, anticatarrhal, antidepressive, anti-inflammatory, cicatrizant, energizing, expectorant, immunostimulant

These small trees, also known as olibanum, grow in north-east Africa and south-east Arabia. Cuts are made in the tree bark from which a white serum exudes, solidifying into "tear drops". When distilled, these produce a pale amber-green essential oil. Frankincense, an ancient aromatic product once considered as precious as gold, has been burnt in temples and used in religious ceremonies since Biblical times.

Frankincense is a gentle oil which is particularly useful for emotional problems, where it allays anger and irritability and soothes grief.

safety
• No known contraindications in normal aromatherapy use.

features in
Beauty and Well-being, The Reproductive Years, The Sunset Years.

△ *Boswellia carteri* – frankincense

△ *Cananga odorata* – ylang ylang

Cananga odorata – ylang ylang
family *Annonaceae*

properties
antidiabetic, antiseptic, antispasmodic, aphrodisiac, calming and sedative, hypotensive, general tonic, reproductive tonic

Ylang ylang trees, with their long, fluttering yellow-green flowers, are native to tropical Asia: ylang ylang is a Malay word meaning "flower of flowers". The blooms are picked early in the morning and steam-distilled to yield an oil with an exotic and heady aroma.

Widely reputed for its aphrodisiac qualities, ylang ylang is said to counter impotence and frigidity. It can help emotional problems such as irritability and fear; and is effective against introversion and shyness. Ylang ylang also helps to regulate cardiac and respiratory rhythm.

safety
• No known contraindications in normal aromatherapy use.
• Use in moderation. Excess can lead to nausea and headaches.

features in
The Teenage Years, Beauty and Well-being, The Sunset Years.

Cedrus atlantica – cedarwood
family *Pinaceae*

properties
antibacterial, antiseptic, cicatrizant, lipolytic, lymph tonic, mucolytic, stimulant

There are 20 or more species of the trees which yield an oil of cedar. This particular tree, the Atlas cedarwood, grows in the Atlas mountains of north Africa. The first oil extracted was used by the Egyptians for embalming. Most of the oil was taken from wood chippings left from making boxes and furniture (King Solomon used cedarwod extensively when building the temple at Jerusalem). Cedarwood oil is now obtained by steam distillation. It has a pleasant, sweet, woody aroma and can be used in a variety of ways.

Cedarwood is effective for oily skin and scalp disorders, and its antiseptic properties and cleansing aroma are beneficial to bronchial problems.

safety
• Unsuitable for pregnant women and small children.
• Should not be taken internally.

features in
The Teenage Years, Beauty and Well-being.

▽ *Cedrus atlantica* – cedarwood

Chamaemelum nobile – chamomile (Roman)
family *Asteraceae*

properties
antianaemic, anti-inflammatory, antineuralgic, antiparasitic, antispasmodic, calming and sedative, carminative, cicatrizant, digestive, emmenagogic, menstrual, vulnerary, stimulant, sudorific

Roman chamomile is native to the British Isles and is a small perennial with feathery leaves and daisy-like flowers. The essential oil is a pale blue-green colour because of the chamazulene content (see *Matricaria recutica* – German chamomile).

The oil is gentle, soothing and calming. It is suitable for children and babies for irritability, inability to sleep, hyperactivity and tantrums. Roman chamomile is also useful for a range of adult complaints, including rheumatic inflammation, indigestion and headaches.

safety
• No known contraindications in normal aromatherapy use.

features in
Beauty and Well-being, The Reproductive Years, The Sunset Years.

△ *Chamaemelum nobile –*
Roman chamomile

△ *Citrus aurantium* var. *amara* – neroli

Citrus aurantium var. amara – neroli
family *Rutaceae*

properties
antidepressant, aphrodisiac, sedative, uplifting

Neroli oil is the distilled oil from the blossoms of the bitter orange tree. It has a soft, floral fragrance, and is the most costly of the orange oils.

Neroli is beneficial for the skin and helps improve its elasticity. It is good for scars, thread veins and the stretch marks of pregnancy and has a sedative and calming effect on the emotions.

safety
• No known contraindications in normal aromatherapy use.

features in
Beauty and Well-being, The Reproductive Years.

Citrus aurantium var. amara – orange (bitter)
family *Rutaceae*

properties
anti-inflammatory, anticoagulant, calming, digestive, sedative, tonic

Oranges have a long tradition in both therapeutic and culinary use. A variety of essential oils are obtained from the fruit, flowers and leaves of both bitter (Seville) and sweet orange trees: neroli oil from the flowers, petitgrain from the leaves, and orange oil from the peel. Bitter orange is expressed from the peel of Seville oranges (most orange marmalades are also made from the peel of Seville oranges).

Bitter orange can be helpful for poor circulation, digestive problems and constipation. It has antidepressant qualities, and will promote positive thinking and cheerful feelings.

safety
• Photosensitizer. Do not expose the skin to sunlight or a sunbed for at least two hours after use.
• No known contraindications in normal aromatherapy use.

features in
The Reproductive Years, The Sunset Years.

△ *Citrus aurantium* var. *amara* –
bitter orange

△ *Citrus aurantium* var. *amara* – petitgrain

Citrus aurantium var. *amara* – petitgrain
family *Rutaceae*

properties
antibacterial, anti-infectious, anti-inflammatory, antispasmodic, calming and energizing

Taken from the leaves of the bitter orange tree, petitgrain's aroma is a cross between the delicate fragrance of neroli oil and the fresh aroma of bitter orange peel. A good petitgrain oil, distilled with some of the blossoms also, is often referred to as the "poor man's neroli" because of its enhanced aroma. Unlike the oil from the fruit, which is expressed, petitgrain oil is obtained by distillation.

Petitgrain is balancing to the nervous system and is recommended for infected skin problems. Emotionally, it can help with anger and panic.

safety
• No known contraindications in normal aromatherapy use.

features in
The Teenage Years.

Citrus bergamia – bergamot
family *Rutaceae*

properties
antibacterial, anti-infectious, antiseptic, antispasmodic, antiviral, calming and sedative, cicatrizant, tonic, stomachic

The main area of bergamot production is southern Italy, although it is also grown on the Ivory Coast. The greenish essential oil is expressed from the peel of this bitter, inedible citrus fruit, which in Cyprus is often crystallized and eaten with a cup of tea. Traditionally, bergamot is a principal ingredient in eau-de-cologne because of its refreshing aroma, and is famous for its use as the flavouring in Earl Grey tea.

Bergamot is useful both in the treatment of digestive problems, such as colic, spasm and sluggish digestion, and for calming emotional states, such as agitation and severe mood swings. It is effective on cold sores but use with extreme caution if in strong sunlight.

safety
• Photosensitizer. Do not expose the skin to sunlight or a sunbed until at least two hours after using.
• Bergapten-free bergamot is an adulterated oil and should not be substituted for the whole essential oil. If not going into the sun, bergamot can be used in the same way as any other oil without risk.

features in
Beauty and Well-being, The Sunset Years.

▷ *Citrus bergamia* – bergamot

△ *Citrus limon* – lemon

Citrus limon – lemon
family *Rutaceae*

properties
antianaemic, antibacterial, anticoagulant, antifungal, anti-infectious, anti-inflammatory, antisclerotic, antiseptic, antispasmodic, antiviral, calming, carminative, digestive, diuretic, expectorant, immunostimulant, litholytic, phlebotonic, stomachic

Lemon juice and peel are widely used in cooking, and the essential oil is expressed from the peel of fruit not sprayed with harmful chemicals. Natural waxes in the oil may appear if it is kept at too low a temperature, but this does not detract from its quality or effectiveness.

Oil of lemon is an underestimated and extremely useful oil. It has an anti-infectious and expectorant effect on the respiratory airways and can help to eliminate the toxins which cause arthritic pain. It is also good for greasy skin. The clean, lively scent can lift the spirits, dispel sluggishness and indecision and relieve depression. Oil of lemon can also help to dispel fear and apathy.

safety
• Photosensitizer. Do not expose the skin to sunlight or a sunbed for two hours after using.

features in
The Teenage Years, Beauty and Well-being, The Reproductive Years, The Sunset Years.

△ *Citrus paradis –*
grapefruit

Citrus paradis – grapefruit
family *Rutaceae*

properties
antiseptic, aperitif, digestive, diuretic

Originating in tropical Asia and the West Indies, the grapefruit tree is now cultivated mainly in North and South America. The yellow oil, produced mainly in California, is obtained by expression of the peel and has a sweet, citrus aroma.

It is effective in caring for oily skin and acne, and regular use twice daily is helpful for cellulite, water retention and obesity. Its antiseptic property is particularly useful in a vapourizer to disinfect the air of a sickroom. It is useful to add a little (4 drops per litre) to spring water when travelling to help prevent digestive problems.

safety
• No known contraindications in normal aromatherapy use.

features in
The Teenage Years, Beauty and Well-being, The Sunset Years.

Citrus reticulata – mandarin
family *Rutaceae*

properties
antifungal, antispasmodic, calming, digestive

The mandarin orange tree originates in China, and its fruit was named after the Chinese Mandarins. The fruit of the mandarin tree is very similar to the tangerine and oils from both fruits may be sold as mandarin. The essential oil is expressed from the peel.

Mandarin oil has digestive properties, and is excellent for treating both adults and children with indigestion, stomach pains and constipation. It can be very useful for over-excitement, stress and insomnia. It is often popular with children because of its gentle action and familiar orangey aroma.

safety
• No known contraindications in normal aromatherapy use.

features in
The Reproductive Years, The Sunset Years.

△ *Citrus reticulata –*
mandarin

△ *Cupressus*
sempervirens –
cypress

Cupressus sempervirens – cypress
family *Cupressaceae*

properties
antibacterial, anti-infectious, antispasmodic, antisudorific, antitussive, astringent, calming, deodorant, diuretic, hormone-like, neurotonic, phlebotonic, styptic

Cypress oil is distilled from the leaves, cones and twigs of the cypress tree. *Sempervirens* is Latin for evergreen, and the resinous wood of this ancient tree has long been used as an aromatic.

The astringent action of cypress oil helps to regulate the production of sebum, reduce perspiration (even of the feet) and to staunch bleeding. It is reputed to help calm the mind where grief is present, and to induce sleep.

safety
• No known contraindications in normal aromatherapy use.

features in
Beauty and Well-being, The Reproductive Years, The Sunset Years.

Eucalyptus smithii – eucalyptus
family *Myrtaceae*

properties
analgesic, anticatarrhal, anti-infectious, antiviral, balancing, decongestant, digestive stimulant, expectorant, prophylactic

Known as gully gum, this tree is native to Australia. The oil distilled from its leaves is equally beneficial to, and much gentler than, the more common *Eucalyptus globulus*, or blue gum, which needs care in use. Because of its gentle action, gully gum eucalyptus is ideal for children; its aroma is also not as piercing as blue gum eucalyptus, which is usually rectified to increase its cineole content.

Eucalyptus is good for muscular pain and is effective against coughs and colds, both as a preventive and as a remedy. *E. smithii* oil has great synergistic power.

safety
- No known contraindications in normal aromatherapy use.
- Keep to the recommended dilution when using as an inhalant for children.

features in:
Beauty and Well-being, The Reproductive Years, The Sunset Years.

△ **Eucalyptus smithii –**
Gully gum eucalyptus

△ **Foeniculum vulgare – fennel**

Foeniculum vulgare – fennel
family *Apiaceae* (or *Umbelliferae*)

properties
analgesic, antibacterial, antifungal, anti-inflammatory, antiseptic, antispasmodic, cardiotonic, carminative, decongestant, digestive, diuretic, emmenagogic, lactogenic, laxative, litholytic, oestrogen-like, respiratory tonic

Fennel is widely grown in the Mediterranean area and the essential oil is distilled from its seeds. The delicate flower heads of all this family resemble umbrellas, as indicated by the original family name, *Umbelliferae*.

Fennel is recommended for lack of breast milk and because it is oestrogen-like, it can be valuable for PMS, the menopause and ovary problems. It will also work efficiently as a diuretic.

safety
- Safe in normal aromatherapy amounts.
- Should not be used during pregnancy before the seventh month.

features in
Beauty and Well-being, The Reproductive Years.

Juniperus communis – juniper
family *Cupressaceae*

properties
analgesic, antidiabetic, antiseptic, depurative, digestive tonic, diuretic, litholytic, sleep-inducing

The juniper tree is a small evergreen from the same family as cypress. The essential oil, distilled from the dried ripe berries (and sometimes the twigs and leaves), has a sweet fragrant aroma. Take care when buying juniper oil, as the berries are used to flavour gin and the residue is often distilled to produce a poor quality essential oil. Even genuine juniper oil can be frequently adulterated.

Juniper oil has a strong diuretic action which is useful for treating cystitis, water retention and cellulite. It has a cleansing, detoxifying action on the skin, and is useful for oily skin problems, such as acne. It is especially good for feelings of guilt and jealousy, and for giving strength when feeling emotionally drained.

safety
- No known contraindications in normal aromatherapy use.
- May be neurotoxic if used without due care and attention.

features in
The Teenage Years, Beauty and Well-being, The Reproductive Years, The Sunset Years.

△ **Juniperus communis –**
juniper

◁ *Lavandula angustifolia* – lavender

Lavandula angustifolia – lavender
family *Lamiaceae*

properties

analgesic, antibacterial, antifungal, anti-inflammatory, antiseptic, antispasmodic, calming and sedative, cardiotonic, carminative, cicatrizant, emmenagogic, hypotensive, tonic

Lavender is the most widely used aromatherapy oil. It is obtained from the plant's flowering tops, and grows wild throughout the Mediterranean region, although it is now cultivated worldwide. In spite of this, it is not easy to find a quality oil. Lavandin, a cheaper oil from a hybrid plant, is often substituted for true lavender.

Lavender is a skin rejuvenator, and helps to normalize both dry and greasy skins. It works in combination with other oils to alleviate arthritis and rheumatism, psoriasis and eczema. It aids sleep, relieves tension headaches, and is good for calming nerves, lifting depression, relieving anger, and soothing fear and grief.

safety

• No known contraindications in normal aromatherapy use.

features in

The Teenage Years, Beauty and Well-being, The Reproductive Years, The Sunset Years.

Matricaria recutica – chamomile, German
family *Asteraceae*

properties

antiallergic, antifungal, anti-inflammatory, antispasmodic, cicatrizant, decongestant, digestive tonic, hormone-like

German chamomile, an annual herb, grows naturally in Europe and its small white flowers are widely used in teas and infusions to aid relaxation and induce sleep. When the flowers are distilled a deep blue oil is produced. The blue colour is produced by the presence of chamazulene, a chemical not present in the plant but formed during the distillation process.

Chamazulene, in synergy with the other components of the oil, is a strong anti-inflammatory agent, which is especially useful for skin problems (particularly irritated skin) and rheumatism, when a compress is most effective. The oil is recommended for premenstrual syndrome, and for calming anger and agitated emotional states.

safety

• No known contraindications in normal aromatherapy use.

features in

Beauty and Well-being, The Reproductive Years, The Sunset Years.

△ *Matricaria recutica* – German chamomile

△ *Melaleuca alternifolia* – tea tree

Melaleuca alternifolia – tea tree
family *Myrtaceae*

properties

analgesic, antibacterial, antifungal, anti-infectious, anti-inflammatory, antiparasitic, antiviral, immunostimulant, neurotonic, phlebotonic

The tea tree plant is native to Australia. Traditionally, a type of herbal tea is prepared from its leaves, and the oil has long been recognized by the Australian Aborigines for its powerful medicinal properties.

Essential oil of tea tree has strong antiseptic properties with a matching aroma, and has excellent antimicrobial and antifungal action. It is a powerful stimulant to the immune system. The unadulterated essential oil has been found to be non-toxic and non-irritating to the skin, and is one of the few essential oils that can be applied directly and undiluted on the skin and all mucous surfaces. The antifungal activity of tea tree oil is much used against *Candida albicans*. It is also effective against some viruses, such as enteritis.

safety

• No known contraindications in normal aromatherapy use.

features in

The Teenage Years, Beauty and Well-being.

Melaleuca viridiflora – niaouli
family *Myrtaceae*

properties
analgesic, antibacterial, anticatarrhal, anti-infectious, anti-inflammatory, antiparasitic, antipruritic, antirheumatic, antiseptic, antiviral, digestive, expectorant, febrifuge, hormone-like, hypotensive, immunostimulant, litholytic, phlebotonic, skin tonic

Niaouli trees originate from the region of Gomene in the South Pacific island of New Caledonia, hence "gomenol" became an alternative name. The trees are large with a bushy foliage and yellow flowers. The steam-distilled leaves and young stems yield an essential oil, which has a eucalyptus-type aroma. The majority of the oil is produced in Australia and Tasmania and very little is exported, making the genuine oil hard to find.

Niaouli is useful for a range of problems experienced by women. It is also a powerful antiseptic and anti-inflammatory agent, and is effective for respiratory problems, such as bronchitis and colds. Its properties suggest it will help against grief and anger.

safety
• No known contraindications, but pregnant women and children should use with care.

features in
Beauty and Well-being, The Reproductive Years, The Sunset Years.

◁ *Melaleuca viridiflora –* niaouli

△ *Melissa officinalis –* melissa

Melissa officinalis – melissa
family *Lamiaceae*

properties
anti-inflammatory, antispasmodic, antiviral, calming and sedative, choleretic, digestive, hypotensive, sedative, capillary dilator

Melissa, also known as lemon balm, is a small herb with tiny, white flowers originating from southern Europe. A daily drink of tea prepared from the fresh leaves is supposed to encourage longevity. The distilled yield from the leaves is tiny, making it a very expensive oil. Much of the melissa oil sold commercially is blended with cheaper essential oils and achieves a similar aroma.

Melissa's sedative action relieves headaches and insomnia and is particularly beneficial for a problematic menstrual cycle. It is also a tonic for the heart, calming the turbulent emotions of grief and anger and helping to relieve fear.

safety
• Photosensitizer. Do not expose the skin to sunlight or a sunbed for two hours after using.
• It is difficult to obtain pure melissa oil, and many fakes contain skin irritants.
• No known contraindications in normal aromatherapy use.

features in
Beauty and Well-being, The Reproductive Years, The Sunset Years.

Mentha piperita – peppermint
family *Lamiaceae*

properties
analgesic, antibacterial, antifungal, anti-inflammatory, antimigraine, antilactogenic, antipyretic, antispasmodic, antiviral, carminative, decongestant, digestive, expectorant, liver stimulant, hormone-like, hypotensive, insect repellent, mucolytic, neurotonic, reproductive stimulant, soothing, uterotonic

The peppermint plant has dark green leaves from which its essential oil is distilled. The oil has a strong, refreshing aroma and is used extensively in the food and pharmaceutical industries, particularly for toothpaste, chewing gum and drinks.

Peppermint is renowned not only for its beneficial effect with digestive problems, such as indigestion, nausea, travel sickness, and diarrhoea, but also for respiratory problems. It can help to clear congestion or catarrh and is useful for bronchitis, bronchial asthma, sinusitis and colds. It helps to clear the mind, and will aid concentration and overcome mental fatigue and depression. It is also useful against anger, guilt and apathy. This is a good essential oil to keep to hand in the first aid cabinet.

safety
• Use sparingly and keep to recommended dilution.
• May counteract homeopathic remedies.

features in
Beauty and Well-being, The Reproductive Years, The Sunset Years.

△ *Mentha piperita –* peppermint

Ocimum basilicum var. *album* – basil
family *Lamiaceae*

properties
analgesic, antibacterial, antifungal, anti-inflammatory, antiseptic, antispasmodic, antiviral, cardiotonic, carminative, digestive tonic, nervous system regulator, neurotonic, reproductive decongestant

Basil oil has a distinctive aroma and is distilled from the whole plant. Several varieties of basil, with different chemical composition, grow in warm Mediterranean climes (especially France and Italy), with leaves that vary in both size and colour, from green to a deep purplish red. The preferred variety for aromatherapy is *album*, as it is not likely to have a neurotoxic effect.

Basil is known mainly for its effect on the nervous system. It is a good tonic and stimulant and is helpful in coping with unwanted emotions, such as fear and jealousy. Its analgesic property makes it useful in cases of arthritis. It is also good for muscle cramp. Basil is an effective insect repellent, particularly against house flies and mosquitoes.

safety
• No known contraindications in normal aromatherapy use.
• May be neurotoxic if used without due care and attention.

features in
Beauty and Well-being, The Reproductive Years, The Sunset Years.

◁ *Ocimum basilicum* var. *album* – basil

△ *Origanum majorana* – sweet marjoram

Origanum majorana – *sweet* marjoram
family *Lamiaceae*

properties
analgesic, antibacterial, anti-infectious, antispasmodic, calming, digestive stimulant, diuretic, expectorant, hormone-like, hypotensive, neurotonic, respiratory tonic, stomachic, vasodilator

Sweet marjoram is a popular culinary herb and has a reputation for promoting long life. The plant grows in the Mediterranean regions and has tiny, white or pink flowers: the oil is distilled from the plant's leaves and flowers. Sweet marjoram should not be confused with the sharp-smelling Spanish marjoram (*Thymus mastichina*), which is a species of thyme.

Sweet marjoram has been shown to be antiviral and is useful for cold sores. It can ease tension and irritability, lift headaches (especially those connected with menstruation) and promote sleep. It is useful for grief and anger, and its ability to calm and uplift makes it useful to combat moodiness.

safety
• No known contraindications in normal aromatherapy use.

features in
Beauty and Well-being, The Reproductive Years, The Sunset Years.

Pelargonium graveolens – geranium
family *Geraniaceae*

properties
analgesic, antibacterial, antidiabetic, antifungal, anti-infectious, anti-inflammatory, antiseptic, antispasmodic, astringent, cicatrizant, decongestant, digestive stimulant, haemostatic, styptic, insect repellent, phlebotonic, relaxant

The geranium plant is cultivated in Egypt, Morocco, the Reunion Islands and China. The oil is distilled from the aromatic leaves, the aroma of which depends on the variety of the plant and where it is grown. Some geranium oils have a definite rose-like smell and are often referred to as rose geranium. More correctly, rose geranium is when a tiny percentage of rose otto is added to the geranium oil.

Geranium will reduce inflammation and is good for acne, herpes, diarrhoea and varicose veins. It is also a relaxant, and will help grief and anger. It is useful for general moodiness and to balance the mood swings associated with PMS.

safety
• No known contraindications in normal aromatherapy use.

features in
The Teenage Years, Beauty and Well-being, The Reproductive Years, The Sunset Years.

◁ *Pelargonium graveolens* – geranium

△ *Pinus sylvestris* – pine

Pinus sylvestris – pine
family *Pinaceae*

properties
analgesic, antibacterial, antifungal, anti-infectious, anti-inflammatory, antisudorific, balsamic, decongestant, expectorant, hormone-like, hypotensive, litholytic, neurotonic, rubefacient

Pine-needle essential oil has a warm, resin-like aroma and is distilled from the Scots-pine tree, which grows widely throughout Europe and Russia.

Pine is an excellent disinfectant and air-freshener: when dispersed in the air, its antiseptic qualities help to prevent the spread of infections. It is recommended for respiratory tract infections and hay fever, while its anti-inflammatory action makes it useful for cystitis and rheumatism. Pine is an excellent pick-me-up for general debility and lack of energy, and is said to dispel melancholy and pessimism.

safety
• No known contraindications in normal aromatherapy use.

features in
Beauty and Well-being, The Reproductive Years, The Sunset Years.

Pogostemon patchouli – patchouli
family *Lamiaceae*

properties
antifungal, anti-infectious, anti-inflammatory, aphrodisiac, cicatrizant, decongestant, immunostimulant, insect repellent, phlebotonic

The plant grows mainly in East Asia and its essential oil has a soft, balsamic aroma. The leaves are cut every few months as the newest ones yield the most oil. Patchouli oil improves with age and has a musty, exotic aroma that is very penetrating.

Patchouli is particularly valuable for broken, chapped and cracked skin, as well as inflamed skin, eczema and acne. It promotes the growth of new skin cells, which makes it helpful in reducing scar tissue. It is beneficial against haemorrhoids and varicose veins. It has a sedative effect on the emotions; its anti-inflammatory property helps calm anger and its antifungal property is useful for jealousy. It is said to help soothe an overactive mind.

safety
• No known contraindications in normal aromatherapy use.

features in
Beauty and Well-being, The Reproductive Years.

▷ *Pogostemon patchouli* – **patchouli**

△ *Rosa damascena* – rose otto

Rosa damascena – rose otto
family *Rosaceae*

properties
antibacterial, anti-infectious, anti-inflammatory, astringent, cicatrizant, neurotonic, sexual tonic, styptic

The much-prized rose otto, also known as attar of roses, is distilled from the deep pink rose petals of this flowering shrub. The genuine, pure oil is extremely expensive as the petals contain very little oil. Roses for distillation are cultivated chiefly in Bulgaria, Turkey and Morocco. Rose absolute is extracted from the petals by a different process, and is a cheaper oil.

Rose otto has been favoured by women through the ages for its gentle action and fragrant aroma. It is said that rose otto balances the hormones and that it is helpful for irregular periods. Rose soothes the skin, lifts depression, and calms inflamed emotions, promoting feelings of happiness and well-being.

safety
• No known contraindications in normal aromatherapy use.

features in
Beauty and Well-being, The Reproductive Years, The Sunset Years.

▷ *Rosmarinus officinalis –* rosemary

Rosmarinus officinalis – rosemary
family *Lamiaceae*

properties
analgesic, antibacterial, antifungal, anti-infectious, anti-inflammatory, antispasmodic, antitussive, antiviral, cardiotonic, carminative, choleretic, cicatrizant, venous decongestant, detoxicant, digestive, diuretic, emmenagogic, hyperglycaemic, blood pressure regulator, litholytic, cholesterol-reducing, mucolytic, neuromuscular effect, neurotonic, sexual tonic, stimulant

Native to the Mediterranean region, rosemary has a long history of culinary and medicinal use. This oil, with an impressive list of helpful properties, is obtained from the pale-blue flowers of the aromatic plant.

Rosemary is helpful for respiratory problems, arthritis, congestive headaches and constipation. It is also a tonic for the liver. This oil stimulates both body and mind. It lifts depression, clears the mind, and is an excellent memory aid.

safety
No known contraindications in normal aromatherapy use.

features in
The Teenage Years, Beauty and Well-being, The Reproductive Years, The Sunset Years.

Salvia sclarea – clary sage
family *Lamiaceae*

properties
antifungal, anti-infectious, antispasmodic, antisudorific, decongestant, detoxicant, oestrogen-like, neurotonic, phlebotonic, regenerative

The strong smelling essential oil of clary sage is distilled from the dried clary sage plant and is used in eau-de-cologne, lavender water, muscatel wines and vermouth. It should not be confused with sage oil and is not a substitute for it.

Clary sage is excellent for all menstrual complications; its oestrogen-like qualities make it good for hormonal problems. It encourages menstruation and is useful for the hot flushes of the menopause. Clary sage is helpful for depression and fear, and during general convalescence.

Safety
- No known contraindications in normal aromatherapy use.
- Prolonged inhalation may cause drowsiness.
- Avoid alcohol consumption for a few hours before or after use.

features in
The Teenage Years, Beauty and Well-being, The Reproductive Years, The Sunset Years.

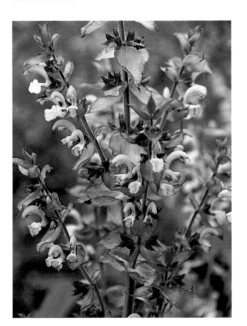

△ *Salvia sclarea –* clary sage

▷ *Santalum album –* sandalwood

Santalum album – sandalwood
family *Santalaceae*

properties
anti-infectious, astringent, cardiotonic, decongestant, diuretic, moisturizing, nerve relaxant, sedative, tonic

The sandalwood tree is native to India, and its cultivation is controlled by the government of that country – for each tree felled, another is planted. The offcuts and wood chips from the sandalwood furniture industry in India, together with the tree roots, are distilled to obtain the essential oil. The sweet, woody aroma of the oil has a soft and therapeutic effect.

Sandalwood, although a gentle oil, is important in the treatment of genito-urinary infections, especially cystisis. It is used for its effect on the digestive system, relieving heartburn and nausea, including morning sickness. It has been found to benefit both acne and dry skin (including dry eczema), as well as being useful for haemorrhoids and varicose veins. Its tonic properties are thought to be helpful in cases of impotence. Sandalwood can also be useful against fear.

Safety
- No known contraindications in normal aromatherapy use.

features in
The Teenage Years, Beauty and Well-being, The Reproductive Years, The Sunset Years.

Thymus vulgaris – thyme, sweet
family *Lamiaceae*

properties
antifungal, anti-infectious, anti-inflammatory, antiseptic, antispasmodic, antiviral, diuretic, immunostimulant, neurotonic, sexual tonic, uterotonic

Thyme is native to the Mediterranean region and is a well-known culinary herb. The essential oil is distilled from its leaves and tiny purplish flowers. There are many different varieties of thyme oil, some of which need careful handling. The alcohol chemotypes of thyme (linalool and geraniol) are the safest for general use.

Sweet thyme is useful for respiratory problems, infections, and digestive complaints. It is especially helpful for insomnia of nervous origin. Sweet thyme is a safe, uterotonic oil to use towards the end of pregnancy and during labour, and it is known to facilitate delivery.

safety
• No known contraindications in normal aromatherapy use.

features in
Beauty and Well-being, The Sunset Years.

▷ *Thymus vulgaris –*
sweet thyme

△ *Zingiber officinale –*
ginger

Zingiber officinale – ginger
family *Zingiberaceae*

properties
analgesic, anticatarrhal, carminative, digestive stimulant, expectorant, general tonic, sexual tonic, stomachic

This perennial herb is native to the tropical parts of Asia. The root, which is used in cooking, is renowned for its heat and for its digestive properties. Its yellow oil is distilled from the roots and, although it has a spicy aroma, the heat does not come through into the essential oil during distillation.

Ginger essential oil has properties which alleviate most digestive problems, including flatulence, constipation, nausea and loss of appetite. Its ability to dull pain is beneficial to muscular pain and sciatica, while its tonic properties are useful for emotions like fear and apathy, and will also help to draw out a reticent, withdrawn personality.

safety
• No known contraindications in normal aromatherapy use.

features in
The Reproductive Years, The Sunset Years.

Special essential oils

Myristica fragrans – nutmeg
Pimpinella anisum – aniseed
Salvia officinalis – sage
Syzygium aromaticum – clove bud

There are some highly beneficial, but very powerful oils which are recommended in this book for special use only. These are used in pregnancy to facilitate delivery. However, their use is not advised without training in aromatherapy or aromatic medicine.

safety
• These oils must only be used in the manner and amounts advised.
• Always seek advice from a qualified aromatherapist before home use.

featured in
The Reproductive Years.

◁ *Myristica fragrans –* **nutmeg**

▷ *Syzygium aromaticum –* **clove bud**

◁ *Salvia officinalis –* **sage**

Aromatherapy
Techniques

Gentle, simple application techniques mean

that aromatherapy can be used safely at home

by women of all ages. Essential oils can be used

in baths, drinks, inhalations, gargles, vaporizers,

compresses and massage for complete beauty and

well-being treatments.

Using inhalations and baths

Essential oils are rarely used in their original, concentrated form but are always taken into the body via a carrier substance. This can be anything which takes the oils into the body: air, water, vegetable oils, lotions and creams are all carriers.

inhalation

When we breathe in the fragrance of an essential oil, some of its molecules travel to the lungs, pass through the lining and into the bloodstream, where they travel around the body. Other molecules take an upward route to the brain, which receives a healing message – to relax or energize, for example – and transmits the appropriate signal along the nerve channels of the body.

Inhalation is the quickest way for oils to enter the body, and is the most effective way to deal with fragile emotions, and negative states of mind such as stress and depression. It is very useful for respiratory conditions, especially those that may present an emergency situation, such as bronchitis or asthma Although essential oils may be inhaled directly from the bottle, other methods are preferred.

△ **A few drops of lavender oil, added to a tissue and sniffed throughout the day, can relieve headaches**.

the hands

This method is useful for emergencies. Put one drop of essential oil into your palm and rub your hands briefly together. Now cup your hands over your nose, avoiding the eye area, and take a deep breath.

a tissue

Place a few drops of essential oil on to a tissue and take three deep breaths. The tissue can then be placed on your pillow or inside your shirt, so that you will continue to benefit from the oil's aroma.

steam inhalation

Fill a basin with hot water and add no more than 2-3 drops (use 1-2 drops for children and the elderly) of essential oil. Keeping your eyes closed to protect them from the powerful vapours, lower your head over the bowl and breathe in deeply.

a vaporizer

This is one of the most popular methods of all for oil inhalation. Electric vaporizers are available, and are the safest types to use. Night-light vaporizers (or oil burners) are inexpensive and readily available in different sizes and designs. The basic model involves a night-light candle standing under a tiny

◁ **Using an oil burner is a popular way of vaporizing essential oils. Keep enough water in the top to stop it drying out.**

▷ **A steam inhalation using eucalyptus oil can help to relieve head colds and sinus congestion.**

△ **Dry skin will benefit from an essential oil mix: it is best massaged on to your body after a bath.**

cup filled with water, to which a few drops of oil are added. Keep the vaporizer out of the reach of children and pets. Top up the water and add more oils as necessary.

Use a vaporizer to keep infections at bay, to relax after a stressful day, or to set the mood for a party or a romantic evening. The number of oil drops is not critical and really depends on the size of the room.

safety

•The quantities of essential oils given above for inhalations are suitable for children and the elderly unless otherwise stated.

bathing

Essential oils do not dissolve well in water, and it is important that the molecules are evenly distributed. Bathing can enhance the effects of essential oils: the oils are not only absorbed through the skin but their aroma is also inhaled. There are several ways to enjoy bathing with essential oils.

bath

Run the water in the bath to a comfortable temperature. Next, add 6–8 drops of oil, then swish the water thoroughly to disperse

▷ **Pamper yourself and unwind with a relaxing aromatherapy bath at the end of a tiring day.**

the oil. Sit in the bath, and for maximum benefit, stay in the water for at least ten minutes to allow the oil to penetrate your skin and to enjoy the benefits of its aroma.

If you prefer, the oils can be mixed with 15 ml/1 tbsp dairy cream or honey before being added to the bath. This will help to disperse the oils. Alternatively, you can mix the oils into powdered milk, adding water to make a paste, before adding the mixture to the bath water. Bath oil prepared from vegetable oil and mixed with essential oils is fine for dry skin, but will feel greasy on normal skins.

foot and hand bath

For sprains, localized swelling, bruising, or similar general discomforts, ten minutes in a foot or hand bath containing 6–8 drops of your chosen oils will bring welcome relief. Remember to keep a kettle of warm water nearby to add to the water in the bowl before it cools too much for comfort.

sitz–bath

For vaginal thrush, a sitz–bath with essential oils is an effective treatment. Fill a large bowl one-third full with warm water and add 3–4 drops of your chosen oil. Sit in the bath for ten minutes.

showers

It is not as easy to benefit from essential oils in the shower. However, you can add some oils to your shower gel or put some on to a sponge. Rub this over your body in the shower, or before you get into it. Make the most of the aroma, breathing deeply and rubbing with your sponge or hands while slowly rinsing. If you wash off the oils too quickly, you won't feel the benefit. Finish with a body lotion mixed with an oil.

safety

•For children and the elderly the essential oil quantities should be halved.

Using compresses, gargles and drinks

Further effective ways of carrying essential oils into the body, using water as the carrier, are with compresses, gargles, mouthwashes and drinks. For the latter, it is important that the essential oils used, and the number of drops, are exactly as recommended.

compresses

A compress brings effective relief in cases such as insect bites, arthritic joints, period or stomach pain, headache, sprains and varicose veins. Use a cold compress if there is inflammation and/or heat, and a warm compress if there is pain or a dull ache.

To make the compress, you need a piece of clean material and a container of water. Soft cotton or linen are the best materials to

▽ A compress is a simple way to use essential oils, and the result can be very soothing.

use. The container should be big enough to hold just enough water to soak into the compress: for example, an egg cup will be big enough for a finger compress, and a small bowl is suitable for an abdomen compress. Add your chosen essential oils to the water: 2 drops of oil is enough for a finger compress, and up to 8 drops of oil is enough for larger body compresses.

Stir the water in the container to disperse the essential oils, then gently lower the compress material on top to allow it to absorb the oils. When the material is wet, squeeze it lightly, position it on the area to be treated, and cover with cling film (plastic wrap) to hold it firmly in place.

For a cold compress, place a sealed, plastic bag of frozen peas or crushed ice cubes over the treatment area and hold in place. For a warm compress, wrap a strip of material such as a scarf, thermal garment or a small towel around the cling film. To keep a compress in place on an arm or leg, an old sock or pair of tights is ideal. Leave the compress in place for at least an hour, or overnight for a septic wound.

gargles and mouthwashes

For sore throats, voice loss and colds which may go on to the chest, gargling with one or more essential oils can be very helpful. Put 2-3 drops of antibacterial essential oils into a glass and half-fill with water. A drop of a soothing oil can also be added. Stir well, take a mouthful, gargle and spit out. Stir again and repeat. It is important to stir the mixture before each mouthful so as to redisperse the oils. Gargling should be done twice a day for best results.

The procedure for mouthwashes is the same as for gargling, except that the liquid is swished around inside the mouth (rather than at the back of the throat) for 30 seconds before spitting out.

▷ Adding a few drops of an antibacterial oil to a glass of water makes an effective gargle mix.

△ When using a mouthwash, make sure the oils are well stirred in the water before each sip.

safety

• For children and the elderly the essential oil quantities should be halved.

drinks

To use essential oils in drinks, the oils must be organic and mixed in a suitable carrier.

▷ Organic plants are grown without the use of chemicals. When taking oils internally, it is important to use only those of therapeutic and certified organic quality.

You are advised first to consult a qualified aromatologist or an aromatherapist working alongside a medical doctor. If you wish to use essential oils in water or tea at home without taking professional advice, it is imperative that the essential oils, and the dosage and time scales recommended in this book are strictly adhered to.

water

Drinking plenty of water is good for us. If you are not fond of water as a drink, put 2 drops of an essential oil such as lemon or orange into 1 litre (1¾ pints) of water in a bottle and shake well. For a healthy digestive system, use 1 drop each of peppermint and fennel oil and mix as before. Shake the bottle before drinking. In conjunction with healthy eating habits, 1 drop each of grapefruit and/or cypress, used as before, can help weight loss as part of a slimming and exercise programme.

teas

Only aromatologists are able to prescribe essential oils for internal, medicinal use. Tea is not a medicine, however, but a pleasant drink. If the tea tastes too strong when the oils are added, dilute it with more water.

Tannin-free china tea or rooibos (red bush) tea make the best bases. Put 2–3 drops of essential oil on to the tea leaves or tea bag, add 1 litre (1¾ pints) of hot water, stir well, then remove the tea leaves or bag. The tea will taste better without milk. Never pour essential oil directly into tea: it will be too strong, and the oils will not disperse. Any tea not drunk immediately can be stored in the fridge and reheated as necessary.

For digestive disorders, a cup of tea drunk two or three times a day is a very gentle and effective remedy. Common

◁ Teas made with essential oils can be a pleasant way of enjoying the healing properties of plants.

urinary tract problems, such as cystitis, respond well, as do insomnia and pain from arthritic joints.

safety

- Use only organic essential oils of therapeutic quality for adding to drinks.
- Absolutes or resins should never be ingested.
- These methods should not be used on children, but are suitable for the elderly.
- Never put essential oils directly into a cup of tea or glass of water. Otherwise, the drink will taste far too strong and will be very unpleasant. The oils should be used only by the methods stated.

Aromatherapy massage techniques

Touch is the most basic human impulse, and massage is a therapeutic extension of touch dating back to ancient times. Hippocrates said that "rubbing loosens a joint that is too rigid", and when we hurt ourselves, our first reaction is to rub the pain away.

To experience a massage under qualified and caring hands is a relaxing experience in itself and it can only be enhanced by the addition of essential oils. If you cannot have treatment by a professional aromatherapist, there are some simple massage techniques you can practise at home on yourself or on a partner, using essential oils for beneficial results. In the following pages are three simple self-massage techniques together with useful tips for blending essential oils at home.

Neck and shoulder treatment

Day-to-day stresses and anxieties often manifest themselves as tension in the neck and shoulder muscles, and treating this area can bring immediate benefits. One of the best times to work on your neck and shoulders is just before going to bed, especially if stress or insomnia are a problem. This will help to relax you and will put your body into a healing mode. Prepare your choice of essential oils with a carrier lotion or oil (*see* Preparing Oils for Application). Wear loose clothing or a towel and remove all jewellery for comfort. Apply a little of the oil mix to both shoulders and begin the massage.

△**1** Resting the whole of your relaxed hand gently over the point of your opposite shoulder, move your hand firmly along the top of the shoulder until you reach the neck, then return to the shoulder point. Repeat this circle several times.

◁ **2** Keeping your hand in this position (palm on collarbone and fingers on shoulder muscle), feel with your fingers for any hard tension spots along the muscle and apply firm circular pressure to these with the pads of your three middle fingers. Be careful not to exceed an acceptable pain threshold.

◁ **3** Take your fingers up your neck, repeating the circular movements with your three fingers where there are painful nodules. Repeat steps 2 and 3 if the area is still painful, and finish with several firm circles, as in step 1. Repeat the massage on the opposite shoulder, using your other hand.

Headache treatment

It is instinctive to rub your temples or forehead when you have a headache. Giving yourself a head massage with one or more appropriate essential oils in a carrier lotion or oil can make the massage more effective.

△ **1** Dab a little of the essential oil mix on your fingertips and place your fingers and thumbs at the temples. Place the length of your fingers on to your forehead and move them firmly from the centre towards the temples, returning back to the centre. Repeat several times.

△ **2** Keeping your thumbs in the same position, make circular movements from the centre of the top of your forehead to the upper temple, using only the cushions of your three middle fingers.

△ **3** Repeat these circles 1 cm (½ in) lower down the forehead, again moving from the centre to the temples. Repeat the circles, doing the last one at eyebrow level. With thumbs positioned as before, "glue" your fingers in the temple hollows and make firm circles which move the skin of the temples over the bone beneath. Repeat step 1.

Scalp treatment

A scalp massage is not only very relaxing, but is also very helpful for anyone who is worried about thinning hair, as it stimulates the hair roots. The roots can become starved of nourishment when the scalp muscle becomes too tight – such as through stress, for example – causing the hair to become thin and weak.

△ **1** Place the thumbs at the top of the ears and "glue" the fingers to the scalp, moving it firmly and slowly over the bone beneath.

◁ **2** Place the hands on another part of the scalp and repeat. Carry on until the whole scalp has been covered. Repeat steps 1 and 2 several times.

Preparing oils for application

Essential oils can be added to a range of carrier bases: vegetable oils, unscented lotion or cream. The choice of base depends on how the mixture is to be used, and is also a matter of personal preference.

types of carrier oil

There are many suitable vegetable oils, each with its own benefit. Unrefined, cold-pressed oils are the best for aromatherapy. The basic oils are widely available, while special and macerated oils are available from suppliers. As a guide, use 15–20 drops of essential oil in 50 ml of the base oil for mixtures to be applied to the skin. Reduce the ratio to 1:10 for preparations to be used on the face.

basic oils
Sunflower *Helianthus annuus*
This oil is taken from the seeds of the giant yellow sunflower. It can relieve eczema and dermatitis, lower blood cholesterol, soothe rheumatism, and ease leg ulcers, sprains and bruises. It may also have diuretic properties.

△ **Apply one or two drops of neat essential oil direct to the skin to soothe cuts, bites and stings.**

Sweet almond *Prunus amygdalis* var. *dulcis*
Almond oil is taken from the kernel of the almond nut, but it is difficult to obtain cold-pressed almond oil. This oil alleviates inflamed and irritated skin, helps to relieve constipation, lowers blood cholesterol, and is good for eczema, psoriasis and dry skin.

special oils
These can all be used alone or as 25 per cent of a basic carrier oil.

Evening primrose *Oenethera biennis*
Yellow evening primrose flowers open at dusk, one circle of flowers at a time. The flowers open so quickly that the buds can be watched as they open. The flowers' seeds are cold-pressed when the stem has finished flowering. Evening primrose oil will relieve arthritis, lower blood cholesterol, help PMS, and soothe wounds. It is excellent for eczema, psoriasis and dry skin, and is said to have a beneficial effect on wrinkles.

Hazelnut *Corylus avellana*
Cold-pressed hazelnuts yield an amber coloured oil. Hazelnut oil has astringent properties and can be used to relieve acne, stimulate circulation and protect against the harmful effects of the sun.

Jojoba *Simmondsia chinensis*
Jojoba is not an oil but a liquid wax, which gives it excellent keeping qualities. Jojoba is an analgesic with anti-inflammatory properties, and it will soothe arthritis and rheumatism, acne, eczema, psoriasis, dry skin and sunburn. Jojoba is good for the scalp, and is a useful addition to shampoo.

Rose hip *Rosa canina*
These small berries produce a syrup, a rich source of Vitamin C, and a golden-red oil. Rose hip oil is anti-aging and will help to regenerate tissue. It softens mature skin, and is good to use for burns, scars and eczema.

△ **Essential oils can be added to cold spring water to make your own customized skin toner. Choose the right oils for your skin type.**

macerated oils
The process of macerating (soaking) plants in olive or sunflower oil enhances base oils with the plants' therapeutic properties. These macerated carrier oils can be added to a base vegetable oil, lotion or cream to enrich it. Macerated melissa and lime oils can also be used to enrich base oils.

Calendula *Calendula officinalis*
Often referred to as marigold (although it is not related to French marigold, *Tagetes minuta*), Calendula has anti-inflammatory and astringent properties, and can relieve broken and varicose veins. Apply directly in undiluted form to ease sprains and bruises.

St John's wort *Hypericum perforatum*
With its analgesic and anti-inflammatory properties, St John's wort will help to relieve haemorrhoids, sprains, bruises and arthritis, and can heal burns, sunburn and wounds.

carrier lotion and cream

Unperfumed lotion, which is made from emulsified oil and water, can be used instead of vegetable oil as a carrier base. Lotion is particularly good for all self-application techniques as it is non-greasy. Use a cream if a base richer than a lotion is needed.

To prepare a blend for use on the body, mix 15–20 drops of essential oil with 50 ml (2 fl oz) of lotion or cream. For a blend to be used on the face, mix 5 drops of essential oil per 50 ml (2 fl oz) lotion or cream. Always ensure the jar or bottle you are using for your blend is completely clean and dry.

safety note

Use only half the specified quantity of essential oils in any base carrier – vegetable oil, lotion or cream – if the mixture is to be used on children and the elderly. Pregnant women should always consult a qualified practitioner before using essential oils.

Preparing a blend for the body using vegetable oil

Vegetable oils are excellent carriers for massage. The essential oils readily dissolve in them, and they allow the hands to move continuously on the skin without dragging or slipping. Mineral oil, such as baby oil, is from a mineral, not a vegetable source. It aims to protects the skin by keeping moisture out and will not allow essential oils to penetrate: it is not suitable as a base oil.

ingredients
- essential oils
- vegetable carrier oil

equipment
- screw-top bottle
- label and marker pen

tips

Care should be taken not to use too much of the mixed oil as it can stain sheets and clothes. To stop too much oil coming out at a time, place your fingers over the top of the bottle, tipping it against them. Apply the fingers to the area to be treated, repeating only if you need more oil.

△ **1** Pour 15–20 drops of your chosen essential oil or oils into a 50 ml (2 fl oz) screw-top bottle.

△ **2** Fill the bottle to within 2 cm (¾ in) of the top with your chosen vegetable carrier oil. Use a funnel, if preferred, to avoid any unnecessary spillage.

△ **3** Screw on the top and label the bottle with the quantity of each oil used, what the mixture is to be used for, your name and the date.

Preparing a blend for the body using lotion

A bland, non-greasy lotion is preferable to oil as it is less messy and is absorbed quickly by the skin. A lotion base is better for self-application techniques, as a vegetable oil bottle will become greasy and can easily slip through your fingers.

ingredients
- bland white lotion
- vegetable oil (optional)
- essential oils

equipment
- screw-top jar or bottle
- label and marker pen

tips

Prepare a blend with a cream base in the same way. For a preparation to use on the face, mix 50 ml (2 fl oz) of the base lotion or cream with only 5 drops of your chosen essential oil.

△ **1** For a lotion to use on the body, fill a 50 ml (2 fl oz) jar or bottle three-quarters full with an unperfumed white lotion, or a lotion mixed with a little vegetable oil, if preferred.

△ **2** Add 15–20 drops of the chosen essential oil or oil blend. Screw on the top and shake thoroughly. Add the rest of the lotion but do not fill right to the top, to allow room for reshaking.

△ **3** Screw the top on firmly and shake again. Label with the contents, use, your name and the date. For a facial lotion, mix 50 ml (2 fl oz) of the base lotion with 5 drops of essential oil.

The Teenage Years

Adolescence is a time of change, both physically and emotionally. Aromatherapy can help smooth the transition from childhood to becoming a young woman with gentle cleansing applications and soothing inhalations.

Aromatherapy in adolescence

The actual rate at which children grow up varies greatly and there can be several years difference in the age at which individual children reach puberty. With the advent of puberty, both health and emotional patterns begin to change. The pituitary gland, responsible for the body's physical growth, begins to release hormones which stimulate the ovaries or testicles to produce eggs or sperm. As soon as these hormonal changes begin to take place, the girl starts to become a young woman and the boy a young man.

For a girl, one of the more obvious signs of becoming a young woman is marked by her developing breasts and by the onset of her periods. This can be a difficult time as she either adjusts to the physical changes that are taking place, or worries because they are happening too fast or not fast

ESSENTIAL OILS AND THE SKIN

hair

pore

sebaceous gland

blood vessels

hair follicle

sweat glands

nerve

△ **A basic understanding of how the skin operates will help you to take care of it.**

enough. Essential oils can be extremely useful to alleviate some of the physical discomforts and emotional aspects often associated with puberty and menstruation (*see* The Reproductive Years).

▷ **Being a teenager is not always easy. Hormone imbalances can lead to extreme mood swings and problems with both the hair and the skin.**

The teenage years are typically turbulent times. A girl's body is rapidly growing and changing in new and startling ways, and her hormones are likely to be affecting both her body and her mood. Hormonal changes trigger an imbalance of sebum in the skin (usually increasing the amount produced), which can lead to greasy skin and hair. This can be awkward at a time when a young woman is becoming aware of her appearance, and of the effect she has on the opposite sex, and feelings of inadequacy are common. The associated emotions of anxiety, resentment, fear and jealousy can all increase stress levels and trigger further reactions in the hair, skin and/or nails.

Essential oils can be very useful both in alleviating unsettled emotional states and treating the skin and hair problems themselves. Aromatherapy, used correctly, forms just one part of a holistic approach to health, and this approach should take into account the girl's nutrition and lifestyle habits, as well as any stressful or worrying external circumstances or events in her life, before the essential oils can be chosen. Now that she is no longer a child, a teenager needs to feel in control of her life, and looking after her health is a good way to begin.

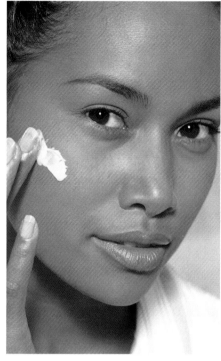

◁ Receiving a shoulder masage is a pleasant and effective way of relieving stress and tension in the neck and shoulders. Ask a friend to gently rub and knead any knotty or tight areas.

△ Experiment with adding oils to your own skin creams and see which combinations work best.

stress and anxiety

Apart from the changes taking place within her own body, life in the outside world can also be problematic for today's teenager. External circumstances, which are beyond her control, can be difficult to manage. If a parent changes job, for example, the family may have to move house and area. This means a new school, with a new teacher, and no immediate friends – all at a time when the academic workload is increasing and exams are becoming a reality. School may also be stressful because of bullying. This affects many teenagers, who exist in a perpetual state of fear and feel they are unable to talk to anyone about it.

There may also be problems within the family: heavy arguments between parents, between the teenager and her parents, or between siblings. For example, teenagers may feel rivalry or jealousy towards a brother or sister who seems to be given more of a parent's love and attention, and receives special treats and favours.

In many societies, the divorce rate is increasing and many modern-day children are "shared" between parents. It is debatable whether it is more stressful to the child to live with parents who don't get on and who argue, or to be caught between two homes.

Growing up involves finding out who you are and having your own ideas and opinions. Problems can arise when parents and their teenage daughter don't see eye-to-eye, and angry fights at home become a routine part of life. Teenagers face strong peer pressure to conform to current trends. This usually involves wearing the "right" clothes, and going to the "right" places for entertainment and holidays. All of these things cost money and can cause tension within the family.

Whatever the reason for stress or anxiety there are numerous relaxing essential oils which can help (*see* Coping with Stress and Emotions). These are best used in the bath or, for more immediate results, by inhalation (*see* Aromatherapy Techniques).

△ Now is a good time to start a daily beauty regime and have fun taking care of yourself.

Everyday skincare

Embarrassing and unsightly skin conditions can be improved by following a healthy diet and a regular skin-cleansing routine using suitable products. The important thing is to follow both of these recommendations if you want to see positive, lasting results.

lifestyle changes

A good starting point is to make a record of your dietary intake each day for a week. By studying this, you will be able to make any necessary adjustments. Try substituting fresh fruit for crisps and chocolate, or fresh juices and/or mineral water for carbonated, sugary drinks. At the same time, monitor improvements to your skin.

If you support yourself by taking aroma-therapy baths to relieve stress and follow the skin-cleansing regime below, you should see visible results within a week. If you do not, it may be because the diet and/or care treatments have not been strictly followed.

△ Regularly cleansing and moisturizing your face will keep your complexion at its best.

Remember, too, that acne is often worse just before menstruation, and that teenage acne usually subsides by the early twenties.

problem skin

The hormonal changes of puberty lead to increased production of sebum by the sebaceous glands in the skin. From the normal, peach-like skin of childhood, a young woman may find her skin (particularly on her face) changing in texture. The pores become enlarged and more open and the skin becomes oily – particularly on the forehead and in a "T-panel" leading down the nose and on to the chin. These open pores are a breeding ground for bacteria, leading to spots, pimples and blackheads, which is why a regular and effective skin-cleansing routine becomes so important.

A spotty skin can become a problem if it develops into acne (*Acne vulgaris*). This is a medical condition and requires special care.

Daily skincare routine

To see an immediate improvement to the skin, a five minute skincare routine should be established and carried out twice a day. Essential oils added to unperfumed creams or lotions can be useful for treating difficult skin conditions and to help with the added emotional difficulties of low self-confidence. With perseverance (and improved lifestyle habits), this routine has proved to be extremely effective. Once the skin begins to improve, stress is reduced and a positive, rather than a negative, cycle is created.

△ **1** Cleanse the skin with a light, water-soluble cleansing milk. Make your own by blending 1 drop each of rosemary, lavender and geranium oils into 30 ml (2 tbsp) base lotion. Rinse off with cold water.

△ **2** Make a gentle, purifying mask by adding 2 drops each of cedarwood, juniper and lemon essential oils to 30 ml (2 tbsp) base cream. Apply to face and leave for ten minutes. Rinse off thoroughly with cold water.

△ **3** Add 3 drops each of lemon and geranium oils to 50 ml (2 fl oz) distilled water. Wipe over the face and neck as a tonic. Follow with a moisturizing lotion mixed with 2 drops of hazelnut oil.

▷ The feet are prone to patches of dry, rough skin. Moisturizing your feet on a regular basis will help to keep them smooth and soft.

▽ Drinking plenty of mineral water can vastly improve your overall health and vitality.

teenage acne

Acne is caused when excessive amounts of sebum form a blockage at the skin's surface on the face, shoulders and back. Cysts, blackheads and red pustules develop, which can lead to pockmark scars. It is difficult to improve the skin once these scars appear.

The rise in the incidence and severity of teenage acne seems to be connected with some aspects of today's modern culture.

Insufficient fresh fruit and vegetables in the diet, chemical additives in food, and air pollution all cause a toxin overload which puts extra strain on the body. Taking good care of your skin and body will really help.

tips for healthy skin
- Stick to a suitable daily skincare routine.
- Exercise for half an hour three times a week.
- Eat lots of fresh fruit and vegetables.
- Drink 6–8 glasses of mineral water a day.

△ Regular steam inhalations with juniper can help clear blocked pores or blackheads.

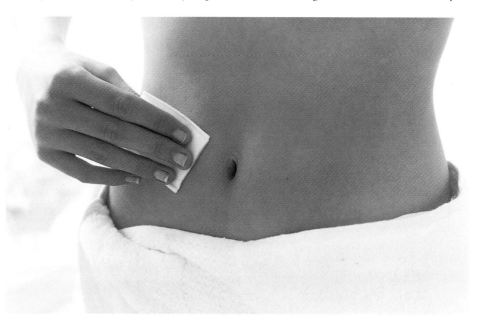

△ Stomach ache or period pains can be treated by applying a compress using basil, lavender and sweet marjoram. A piece of soft cotton or linen soaked in a water-oil mix makes a good compress.

Caring for hair and nails

Both the hair and nails are made of keratin, a modified skin tissue, and both are present to protect us from harm. The hair and nails benefit from good nutrition, and care with essential oils can improve their appearance.

teenage hair

Hair problems for teenagers will often mean greasy hair. Greasy hair needs frequent washing with a suitable shampoo to prevent the excess oil from causing spots around the hairline. However, the rubbing action on the scalp stimulates the sebaceous glands to produce more sebum and can make the problem worse. If you have greasy hair, shampoo it no more than once a day. Add an astringent essential oil to an unperfumed shampoo for your own aromatherapy treatment at home. Take care to apply the shampoo to the hair and not the scalp.

Hair loss can also be a problem for some young women. This can be brought on by the stress of exams and personal worries, and also by harsh treatment of hair that is already weak, such as dragging it back too tightly from the forehead with hairbands. Mixing essential oils with your shampoo can help to strengthen weak hair. Handle hair with care, and ease it forward slightly before adding hairbands and accessories.

conditioning

The condition of our hair is crucial to how we look, and good hair treatment brings its own rewards. Hair should be trimmed regularly – with no more than 1 cm (½ in) removed – to keep the ends strong. This is especially important with long hair: the more often long hair is trimmed, the faster it will grow and the better it will look.

△ **Lavender oil is very useful for treating difficult nail conditions. Add a 2–3 drops to 5 ml (1 tsp) carrier oil and use as required.**

▷ **If your hair lacks lustre, try adding the appropriate oils to an unperfumed conditioner base. After shampooing, gently comb the mix through to the ends of your hair.**

If your hair is in poor condition, use a separate conditioner: products which aim to combine a shampoo with a conditioner are rarely effective as they cannot do both jobs well. Add the essential oils your hair needs to an unperfumed, basic conditioner. Apply the mixture to your hair and scalp after shampooing and towel-drying. Cover with a plastic bag to keep in the heat, and leave for 30 minutes before rinsing well.

tips for healthy hair

• Add 8–10 drops of essential oils to 50 ml (2 fl oz) of unfragranced shampoo (not baby shampoo – it is not especially mild).
• Give yourself a daily scalp massage with soothing essential oils to arrest and prevent early hair loss.

nailcare

Nail-biting is often connected to stress and has a strong emotional component. It can be a difficult habit to break. Because teenage girls are often concerned with appearance, the desire for beautiful, manicured nails may help to overcome the problem.

▷ Strong and beautiful nails begin at the cuticle. Use an oil mix and gently massage it on to the cuticle and surrounding area daily. After three months, you will see improvement in your nails.

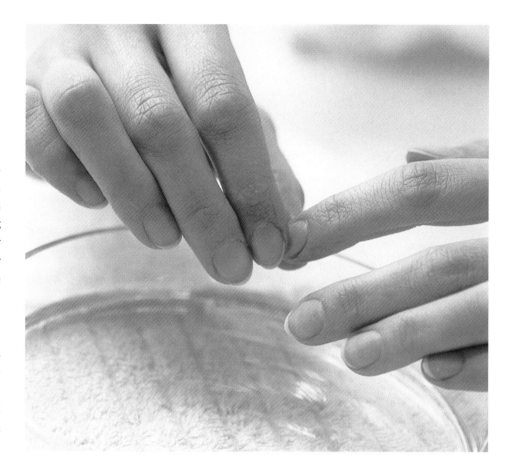

To encourage strong, healthy nails, you have to care for the cuticle as well as the nail, as this is where nail growth begins. Health disorders can cause ridging and thinning of the nails. Psoriasis and fungus under the nail tips can be treated with lavender or geranium oils. As with skin and hair, the nails give an indication of inner health.

tips for healthy nails

• Discourage nail-biting by coating the nails daily with neat lavender oil. The unpleasant taste of the oil will stop the chewing.
• Apply neat lavender oil daily to the nail cuticle to improve the condition of weak nails. Results will show in three months.

Useful essential oils

essential oil	treatment
hair	
Caraway *Carum carvi*	stimulant, encourages hair growth, aids scalp problems.
Cedarwood *Cedrus atlantica*	antiseptic and stimulant to scalp, reduces greasy dandruff, helps to renew hair growth
Clary sage *Salvia sclarea*	regenerative, improves poor hair growth
Juniper *Juniperus communis*	antiseborrhoeic (greasy dandruff), antiseptic (greasy scalp)
Lemon *Citrus limon*	antibacterial, astringent (reduces greasy dandruff)
Rosemary *Rosmarinus officinalis*	stimulating to circulation, helps renew hair growth
Ylang ylang *Cananga odorata*	tonic to scalp, aids hair growth
nails	
Geranium *Pelargonium graveolens*	antifungal (athlete's foot, skin and nail fungi)
Lavender *Lavandula angustifolia*	antifungal (athlete's foot, skin and nail fungi), healing (strengthens weak nails)
Tea tree *Melaleuca alternifolia*	anti-infectious, antifungal (skin and nail infections)

essential oil	treatment
skin	
Geranium *Pelargonium graveolens*	cicatrizant (healing), useful for open acne
Juniper *Juniperus communis*	antiseborrhoeic, antiseptic
Lavender *Lavandula angustifolia*	antiseptic, cicatrizant (healing)
Lemon *Citrus limon*	antibacterial, astringent
Petitgrain *Citrus aurantium* var. *amara* (fol)	anti-inflammatory, antiseptic, useful for infected acne
Cedarwood *Cedrus atlantica*	antiseptic, cicatrizant, stimulant (skin and scalp problems)
stress	
Clary sage *Salvia sclarea*	calming
Geranium *Pelargonium graveolens*	relaxant (agitation, anxiety)
Lavender *Lavandula angustifolia*	calming and sedative
Lemon *Citrus limon*	calming and sedative
Petitgrain *Citrus aurantium* var. *amara* (fol)	balancing and calming
emotions	
Bergamot *Citrus bergamia*	sedative, neurotonic, cicatrizant, antispasmodic (anxiety, agitation, grief, fear, mood swings)

Beauty and Well-being

Aromatherapy works on every level to cleanse the body and balance the mind. Use aromatic essential oils in your daily cleansing and moisturising routines for smoother skin, stronger nails and better-conditioned hair. The healing properties of plants can also play an effective role in stimulating the immune system to strengthen the body against disease.

Looking after yourself

Looking and feeling good is important for most women. Commercial products can do much to treat beauty emergencies, but the only effective, long-term solution is optimum health in body and mind.

beautiful skin

A good complexion is a huge beauty asset: it helps a woman to look good and this, in turn, will boost morale. The skin is the largest organ of the body. It is always on display to the outside world and is worth taking care of. The skin has a slightly acid mantle, which keeps out harmful bacteria, and it is not a good idea to use excessively alkaline cleansers, such as soap, to wash the skin, as these destroy the necessary acid balance. The condition of the skin is a good indicator of general health within the body.

lifestyle

The condition of our skin is affected by our lifestyle and general well-being, including our diet, how much exercise we take, our work, our family and our mental attitude.

△ By carefully placing objects of natural beauty in your home, you can help your mind to relax and unwind. Soft candlelight is traditionally associated with feelings of peace and harmony.

To some extent, we are what we eat. Our circulatory system carries the nutrients from our food around the body: without a healthy diet, the body's cells receive insufficient nutrition. Regular exercise is also important. A sedentary lifestyle, when combined with a lack of exercise, means that food nutrients are not transported around the body efficiently, and toxins in the lymphatic system are not completely eliminated. This can lead to cellulite and other problems in the body and with the skin. A diet which includes plenty of water, fresh fruit and vegetables will help to keep our bodies free from toxins and promote a blooming, clear complexion.

Our day-to-day environment can also affect our bodies. Most homes and offices are centrally heated, and this has a drying effect on skin and hair. Keeping a bowl of water beside each radiator will help to increase humidity. Women who spend a great deal of time outdoors should take care

◁ Strategically placed oil and water mixes can increase humidity levels and also release aromas.

to protect their skin from excessive exposure to the sun, rain and wind: these are all damaging to the skin, and will promote wrinkles and early aging. Protect your skin from exposure to harmful ultraviolet rays, on the sunbed or outdoors, to reduce the risk of skin cancer.

Whether you are a working mother, a full-time mother, or a full-time career woman, feeling happy with what you do is important. This, in turn, is reflected in the condition of the skin, hair and nails. When we are unhappy, we tend to feel negative about ourselves and are more likely to focus on our tiny imperfections. This can leave us feeling even worse and creates a vicious cycle which can lead to depression. With a positive mental attitude, on the other hand, we feel happier and more buoyant, our stress levels decrease, and we look and feel in a healthier state.

the aging process

Like all other organs, the skin deteriorates with age. Typically this is characterized by the slowing down of cell regeneration, and

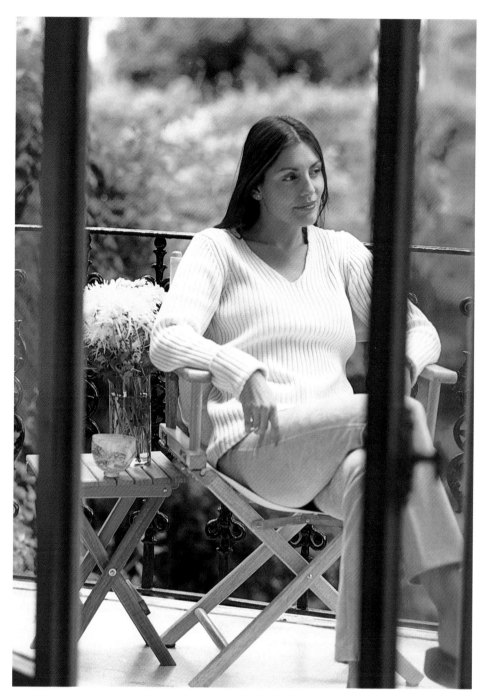

▷ Enjoying some quiet time alone each day is important. It allows you to recharge your batteries, giving you space for relaxation and contemplation without any outside pressures.

the fact that dead skin cells gradually take longer to be discarded. As we grow older, our skin becomes less moist and loses its elasticity. Facial expressions are more likely to develop into wrinkle lines. As oestrogen production decreases during the menopause years (*see* The Sunset Years), there is a thinning and dehydration of the epidermis (the outer layer of the skin).

Many factors play a part in skin aging: heredity, menopause, occupation, exposure to the sun and wind, poor diet, alcohol-consumption, smoking, prolonged stress, insufficient sleep, even crash diets (which can cause wrinkles) and excessive washing (which can dehydrate the skin). The aging process is also partly due to the formation of free radicals in the body, developed from a reaction between sunlight and oxygen. These molecules are unstable and, in their search to stabilize, reactions occur in the body which can cause cellular destruction, resulting in skin aging and internal disease.

Aging is beyond our control, but we can help to minimize its effects by giving our bodies the best attention possible. Lifestyle factors need to be addressed and then supported by a daily care regime

with suitable lotions and creams, which can help to improve the elasticity and appearance of the skin, hair and nails. Protection can be taken against the negative effects of the weather and central heating.

It has been shown that essential oils can be used successfully to combat the effects of aging. Research studies have shown that many essential oils have cell regenerative properties, and essential oil products help to promote a much healthier, younger-looking skin. The essential oil molecules penetrate the skin and are able to work at the germinative layer, where the new cells are formed. These improved cells eventually reach the surface of the skin where the appearance is vastly improved.

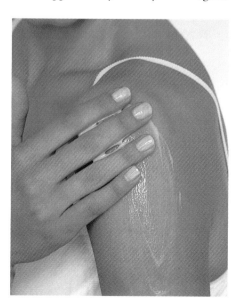

△ Apply a lotion containing analgesic essential oils to relieve aches and pains in the shoulders.

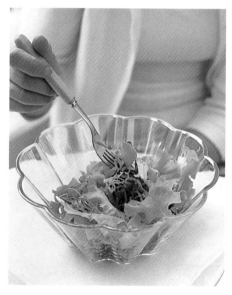

△ Eating plenty of fresh raw vegetables, fruits and salads will keep your energy levels high.

Daily skincare

The sooner a woman begins a good skincare routine, the more she will reap the benefits as she gets older. A good moisturizer is arguably the most important item in a woman's wardrobe – you can replace your clothes, but not your skin. It is well worth investing in an efficient, quality moisturizer that you like to use.

There is a vast array of commercial products available, designed for every skin permutation imaginable: teenage, normal, dry, oily, mature, sensitive, and allergy-prone skins. Although well-formulated cosmetics without essential oils may benefit the skin, a natural, quality range with added essential oils will increase the benefits.

choosing products

With aromatherapy, you should only have to choose between two basic product types because all essential oils are normalizing,

◁ **Always pat your face dry with a soft towel after rinsing. The skin on the face needs careful handling, whatever our age.**

giving exceptional care to the skin. If the skin is normal to oily, then look for a cleansing milk and moisturizing *lotion*. Choose cleansing and moisturizing *creams* when the skin is more dry and in need of nourishment. Look for products which have good quality bases and which don't contain alcohol, lanolin or other animal products. Night creams containing lanolin make your skin greasy, as the molecules are actually too big to penetrate the skin, and the cream will "sit" on top of your face all night, rubbing off on the pillow. Prepare your products with well chosen essential oils in a concentration of 0.5 per cent.

tips for healthy skin

If you wear make-up, it is important to cleanse your skin thoroughly before bed. In the morning, toner on cotton wool (cotton ball) is usually sufficient. Give yourself a treatment mask once a week. After a mask, you should moisturize twice, as masks draw out moisture as well as toxins. If you don't wear any make-up, a mask once a fortnight is usually sufficient.

If you don't wear make-up, use a mild toner only at night-time after cleansing. Moisturize first thing in the morning, after cleansing and toning.

creating your own products

To make your own skincare products, use unperfumed bases, adding the appropriate essential oils, 1 drop for each 10 ml (2 tsp) of carrier. Cold spring water is an excellent basic toner.

oily skin or acne

daytime base lotion with 10 per cent spring water added slowly while stirring.
night-time base lotion with 10 per cent hazelnut oil added slowly while stirring.

△ **Spring water can be used as a basic toner for all types of skin. Add your chosen essential oils.**

dry or mature skin

daytime base lotion with 25 per cent rose hip or jojoba oils added slowly while stirring.
night-time base cream with 50 per cent rose hip or jojoba, or the macerated oils of lime blossom or melissa added while stirring.

at the menopause

Try using hormone-like essential oils such as clary sage and niaouli which both have oestrogen-like properties.

skin disorders

A skin problem can arise from many causes, some of which may be more obvious than others. It may stem from an internal physical problem, such as poor digestion or painful periods, or from a mental problem, such as deep-rooted anxiety or grief. The effects of on-going mental and emotional stress can also cause skin problems, which in turn may aggravate the condition as we become worried, anxious and embarrassed about how others see us.

▷ Roman chamomile is excellent for soothing dry, irritable and inflamed skin. Try adding a few drops to your moisturizer and apply daily.

aromatherapy treatment

Aromatherapy can play an important part in the treatment of skin disorders. The oils are not only able to treat the physical symptoms but, through their aromas, can also affect the mental state of the sufferer. For example, many people suffering chronic, painful skin conditions, such as eczema and psoriasis, may have high stress levels because of the impact of the disease on their physical appearance.

Essential oils are able to break this cycle effectively, lightening the mind as well as tackling the physical symptoms. Where the skin is already being moisturized, whether on the face, hands and/or body, it is easy enough to combine appropriate essential oils with the existing treatment for a two-in-one effect. For example, arthritis oils added to a hand and body lotion base reduce pain and inflammation at the same time as making the skin less dry and scaly.

For severe eczema it is very beneficial to change your diet to one that is dairy-free, eliminating cow's milk and related products from what you eat. This is usually enough to cure the condition, although it can take a few months for the results to be evident. Meanwhile, correct use of the appropriate oils will bring relief from the symptoms.

Acne rosacea, a form of acne which usually attacks women over 30, has similar symptoms to *Acne vulgaris* (*see* The Teenage Years). It seems to affect women who like highly seasoned foods and drink large amounts of tea and coffee. Dietary changes will be highly beneficial in all cases, while the use of aromatherapy treatments will improve the condition of the skin.

Blending essential oils with a moisturizer

For customized skincare, select the appropriate essential oils and add them to a good quality, bland base cream. Add a little rose hip carrier oil if your skin is particularly dry.

ingredients
• 40 ml (8 tsp) unperfumed base cream
• rose hip oil (optional)
• blend of appropriate essential oils

equipment
• small jar
• swizzle stick or teaspoon
• spatula (optional)

tip
Always apply creams to the face with clean hands, and best of all using a spatula, to avoid transmitting germs from your fingernails to the cream, and possibly to your skin.

△ **1** For dry skin, add 5 ml (1 tsp) rose hip oil to a jar containing 40 ml (8 tsp) base moisturizing cream.

△ **2** After blending your own selection of appropriate essential oils, add 5 drops to the moisturizing cream.

△ **3** Stir thoroughly with a swizzle stick or the handle of a clean teaspoon to blend the mixture.

Daily hand, foot and nail care

Our hands are exposed daily to the elements and to household detergents, and our feet carry us wherever we want to go. Both deserve as much attention as the face, and will benefit greatly from aromatherapy.

hand care

It is said that there are two ways to tell a woman's age: by her neck and by her hands. Our hands, like our necks and faces, are always exposed to the air and are always on visible display. However, it is easy to neglect them when leading a busy life.

treatment

Essential oils can be added to a base lotion and used after each time you wash your hands. Patchouli is one of the best oils for cracked, dry skin, and clary sage helps delay cellular aging. If your hands are neglected and in need of a boost, try giving them an exfoliating "mask" treatment before going to bed. After using an exfoliating face mask on your hands, apply your hand lotion. Cover your hands with cling film (plastic wrap) and pull on a pair of cotton gloves, or cotton socks, over the cling film. Keep the mask in place for an hour before rinsing off.

◁ **Having well-cared for hands is a beauty asset. To give your hands a treat, prepare a mix using oils of geranium and rose otto and work well into the skin.**

◁ **For cracked knuckles, try patchouli oil mixed in a carrier cream or lotion base and applied to the affected area on clean, dry hands.**

foot care

Think of the amount of work our feet have to do – we walk on them daily, often in inappropriate footwear, and yet we give them surprisingly little care and attention.

treatment

Spend some time each week giving your feet a thoroughly relaxing massage which benefits your feet and the rest of your body at the same time. Keep them as scrupulously clean as your face, regularly removing dead skin at the heels and drying properly between the toes.

Watch for any broken skin between the toes as this may be an early sign of athlete's foot – a fungal condition which can be difficult to treat once it takes hold. Plastic shoes are a common cause of athlete's foot as they create moisture and cause the feet

to sweat, creating the ideal conditions for fungus to develop. Essential oils can be used to treat all fungus-type infections as well as viral ones, including warts and verrucas. You will also need to address the underlying causes. These may be related to stress and poor nutrition, and will be helped with relaxing essential oils.

nail care

Strong, well-manicured nails on the hands and feet play an important role in a woman's appearance. Brittle, damaged or weak nails can detract from this. Essential oils can be used to improve nail condition.

treatment

Essential oil of lavender is particularly good for strengthening nails. Each evening, put your finger on to the nozzle of a bottle of lavender oil, tip the bottle, and rub the oil into the cuticles. After two or three months you should see some improvement as the treated nail grows through.

△ **Giving yourself a foot massage not only feels good but also energizes the many reflex points on your feet, which in turn correspond to different parts of the body.**

▷ **For tired or swollen ankles, a cool compress soaked in Roman chamomile and lavender oil is both soothing and refreshing and can also alleviate any inflammation.**

Nail treatment

Pampering your nails with this weekly treatment will keep them healthy and strong. If your nails are particularly weak and damaged, you may prefer to apply this quick treatment every evening. Because nail growth is a slow process, the results are not immediate – it will be a couple of months before you see any improvement, but it will be worth the wait.

ingredients
• warm water
• lavender essential oil

equipment
• bowl
• cuticle stick
• cotton bud (Q-tip)

tip
Sucking a jelly cube each day is said to stengthen the nails. If you often have white flecks across your nails, increasing the calcium in your diet could also help.

△ **1** Soak your fingertips in warm water before gently cleaning the surplus cuticle from the nails.

△ **2** Use a cotton bud (Q-tip) to apply neat lavender oil to each cuticle to strengthen them.

Daily bodycare

Our bodies are protected for much of the time with clothes, and because of this, the skin of our torso is usually in a better condition – softer and smoother – than that of our arms and legs, which are more frequently exposed to sunlight.

conditioning treatments

The arms and legs benefit hugely from the daily use of creams and lotions containing essential oils; improvements are particularly apparent when moisturizing bath or shower oils or gels have not been used as a matter of course. If your skin is dry or flaky, put your essential oils into a carrier oil to add a gleam to your skin. (*See* Preparing Oils for Application to select the most beneficial oil for your skin type.)

For a bath treatment for dry skin, grate 15 g (½ oz) unscented, non-alkaline soap into 120 ml (½ cup) boiling water, and stir to dissolve the soap. When cool, add 8 drops of your favourite essential oil or oil mix. Hold your mixture under the running tap to dissolve in the bathwater and make some bubbles. If you prefer lots of bubbles, add essential oils to a non-drying bubble bath.

If you have normal to oily skin, which is not known to be sensitive, give yourself a body rinse before leaving the bath or shower. Dissolve your essential oil or oils into 15 ml (1 tbsp) vodka, and mix with 1 litre (1¾ pints) spring water. Add 120 ml (½ cup) white wine or cider vinegar to the spring water mixture for an extra zingy feel.

If you have a problem with body odour, use the vodka rinse above, but without the vinegar. Add 3 drops of nutmeg essential oil and 3 drops of cypress essential oil; both of these have deodorizing properties.

◁ Varicose veins can be painful and unsightly. A cool compress, made with cypress, clary sage or niaouli oil and applied to the affected area, can help.

For hard, rough skin on elbows and heels, use a facial exfoliating mask, followed by a moisturizing body lotion or oil to which 2–3 drops of essential oil have been added.

Cellulite is caused by ineffective blood circulation, which leads to poor lymphatic drainage and fluid retention. Aromatherapy can help with a daily regime. Pummel the area vigorously before applying essential oils in a carrier lotion or oil.

Varicose vein treatment

Apply the essential oil blend or lotion mix to the whole leg before following the directions below. Upward strokes are important to help the blood move towards the heart. Use phlebotonic oils such as clary sage, cypress and niaouli.

△ **1** Massage the upper half of the leg first with upward movements. This clears the valves to allow the blood to pass more easily from the lower leg.

△ **2** Massage in an upward direction only, using the palms of both hands. Make long, firm strokes alternately with each hand up the calf muscle.

△ **3** Take the fingers of both hands alternately up the calf muscle. Complete the sequence by repeating step 2.

Anti-cellulite treatment

Cellulite is recognized by its resemblance to orange or grapefruit peel. A daily aromatherapy treatment, along with an improved diet and a thorough exercise plan, will boost the circulation and improve lymphatic drainage, helping to disperse the cellulite.

△ **1** After firmly rubbing in your prepared oil mix or lotion, take both hands alternately up the outside of the leg. Use a loofah or bristle brush if preferred.

△ **2** Use the heel of your hands to pummel the cellulite vigorously. This stimulates the circulation and allows quicker penetration of the essential oils.

△ **3** Continue to work over the cellulite area using the heels of both hands alternately. Maintaining the firmness of the strokes, repeat step 1.

Useful essential oils

essential oil	treatment
skin types	
DRY SKIN	
Chamomile (Roman) *Chamaemelum nobile*	anti-inflammatory (irritable skin)
Geranium *Pelargonium graveolens*	anti-infectious, cicatrizant
Lavender *Lavandula angustifolia*	antiseptic, anti-inflammatory, cicatrizant (healing)
Patchouli *Pogostemon patchouli*	anti-inflammatory, cicatrizant
Rose otto *Rosa damascena*	anti-inflammatory (blotchy skin), cicatrizant
OILY SKIN	
Cedarwood *Cedrus atlantica*	antiseptic, antibacterial, cicatrizant.
Lemon *Citrus limon*	astringent, antibacterial, anti-inflammatory
Ylang ylang *Cananga odorata*	tonic, balancing, calming, hypotensive
MATURE SKIN	
Clary sage *Salvia sclarea*	regenerative (cellular aging)
Frankincense *Boswellia carteri*	antioxidant (combats aging process), cicatrizant
anti-aging	
Clary sage *Salvia sclarea*	oestrogen-like, regenerative (counteracts cellular aging)
Frankincense *Boswellia carteri*	antioxidant (combats aging process)
Lemon *Citrus limon*	antisclerotic (combats aging process)

essential oil	treatment
skin conditions	
PSORIASIS (INCLUDING NAILS)	
Bergamot *Citrus bergamia*	cicatrizant
Lavender *Lavandula angustifolia*	cicatrizant
ECZEMA	
Bergamot *Citrus bergamia*	anti-infectious (weeping eczema), cicatrizant
Geranium *Pelargonium graveolens*	analgesic, anti-infectious, anti-inflammatory, cicatrizant
ACNE *ROSACEAE*	
Chamomile (German) *Matricaria recutica*	anti-inflammatory, cicatrizant
Chamomile (Roman) *Chamaemelum nobile*	anti-inflammatory, cicatrizant
Frankincense *Boswellia carteri*	analgesic, cicatrizant
ATHLETE'S FOOT AND NAIL FUNGI	
Clary sage *Salvia sclarea*	antifungal (skin conditions)
Geranium *Pelargonium graveolens*	antifungal, anti-infectious
Lavender *Lavandula angustifolia*	antifungal, antiseptic
CELLULITE	
Cypress *Cupressus sempervirens*	diuretic
Fennel *Foeniculum vulgare*	diuretic, circulatory stimulant
Juniper *Juniperus communis*	diuretic, lypolytic
VARICOSE VEINS	
See The Reproductive Years for relevant essential oils.	

Coping with stress and emotions

There is increasing evidence to suggest that stress features significantly in the lives of many women, whether they are single, married or co-habiting, and whether or not they have children. Many women are finding it increasingly difficult to manage work and home commitments, leisure time and relationships, and these stresses are often multiplied when a woman has children.

Perhaps stress can be defined as having too much to do, in too short a time, and without the necessary resources. When such a situation goes on and on over a period of time, it can have an adverse effect on health. However, when we are unhappy, or under too much pressure for an extended period of time, our body's cells generate a negative, health-reducing effect and stress-related conditions may begin to show: insomnia, tension headaches, chronic back problems, digestive disorders, skin problems and other diseases in the body.

the use of aromatherapy

Essential oils have been proved to have an influence on the central nervous system, which varies depending on the essential oils

△ **Sniffing a tissue prepared with essential oils is a handy method for improving concentration.**

selected. Good use of aromatherapy can improve general health and well-being, helping us to cope with the physical and emotional aspects of stress.

If you are finding it difficult to concentrate on your work, prepare a tissue with a blend

of rosemary and peppermint essential oils, and sniff at intervals throughout the day. Both of these oils are decongestants and mental stimulants, and they should help to clear congested or conflicting thoughts and mixed emotions. Add lemon oil to the blend if you work on a computer. In one Japanese study, it was revealed that 54 per cent fewer typing errors were made by staff who had been exposed to a lemon aroma, compared to those who had not.

TIPS FOR COPING WITH STRESS

- Take regular exercise: join a gym, take up yoga, or go for long walks.
- Put aside some quiet time each day for yourself, for reading, reflection, meditation, visiting friends, or simply doing nothing at all.
- Eat a healthy diet, avoiding snacking on processed foods.
- Devise a schedule at home which means that everyone takes part in running the household.
- If you have a partner, make sure you spend at least one evening a week on your own together.
- Unwind in an aromatherapy bath with a favourite essential oil every evening: this promotes a refreshing sleep, which will help to prepare you for the next day.

emotional insecurity

The emotions we express or feel can be separated into two groups: primary and secondary. Some primary emotions are positive, such as feelings of love, tolerance, and happiness, and these are not a problem. Difficulties arise with the negative primary emotions, such as fear, anger, guilt and

◁ **Inhalation is the fastest way for an essential oil to reach the brain. Vaporize ylang ylang for its balancing and calming properties.**

△ **Basil is useful for its effects on the nervous system**. It can help to dispel fear and jealousy.

jealousy. Secondary emotions are usually concerned with our personality. These may be shown as moodiness, confusion, timidity and inferiority, for example.

Essential oils are very useful for treating emotional problems. The oils are selected on the basis of their properties which relate to the emotion being expressed. For example, essential oils which have relaxing and anti-inflammatory properties are known to be soothing for anger, while oils with stimulating and digestive properties are better able to overcome fear.

anger

The state of anger can range from mild irritability and impatience at one end of the scale to explosive outbursts and fury at the other. The ability to cope with anger varies from person to person, depending on the personality. When under stress, anger is more easily aroused and our ability to deal with our own feelings may be severely tested. It is important to have the ability to handle our anger in a positive, constructive way. The oils which help are, principally, calming, antispasmodic, anti-inflammatory and healing.

fear

Stress and fear are sometimes related, and can be acute or chronic. If you oversleep and are running late for an important meeting, for example, your body goes into a temporary state of fear and your adrenal

glands produce extra adrenalin to help you deal with the situation. However, if the state of fear is long-lasting, it can become a chronic condition that can lead to illness. Living in a state of fear creates tension and anxiety which have a detrimental effect on our outlook and upon our bodies. The helpful essential oils are those which are analgesic, calming and soothing, and those which are stimulating to the mind, as well as to the respiratory and digestive systems.

jealousy

Most jealous feelings are negative. Jealousy is often linked with anger and/or resentment, and may arise out of an inability to share our friends, family and possessions, or else out of a craving for things that we do not have, which other people seem to have. Although jealousy is often the most difficult emotion to admit to, it is one of the most deadly, where we can hurt not only others but also ourselves. Positive thinking and the use of essential oils which will detoxify or destroy fungi and kill viruses can help to overcome this self-destructive emotion.

Secondary emotions can also be helped by essential oils and are sometimes linked with a primary emotion like fear. Lack of confidence or a sense of under-achievement may involve fear, and mood swings may involve anger and/or irritability.

lack of confidence

Many women suffer from a lack of self-confidence. Positive thinking is necessary here, along with neurotonic essential oils which will boost your morale by strengthening the nervous system. These stimulate the mind and will help you to achieve things you never thought were possible. Sweet thyme may help to promote bravery and instil drive and assertiveness due to its many tonic properties. The most effective methods of use are by tissue or vaporizer inhalation, and in the bath.

moodiness

As well as being able to relax or stimulate the nervous system, essential oils can also induce slight mood changes. This makes

▷ **Water with lemon and peppermint can help to dispel apathy and lift feelings of depression.**

△ **A shoulder massage using juniper oil can help when you are feeling emotionally drained**.

the use of essential oils suitable for women who are inclined to be temperamental, and for the unpredictable mood swings and irritability suffered during PMS.

loss of sensual awareness

Feelings of indifference, apathy and general loss of libido can be directly related to stress and/or overwork. Taking an essential oil bath or vaporizing some oils an hour before bedtime will help you to unwind, physically and emotionally. You and your partner may like to give each other aromatherapy back or shoulder massages to help each other relax and to prepare for love-making. Use essential oils which are renowned for their aphrodisiac and uplifting effects.

Common health problems

There are several relatively common health problems which can occur at any age and with varying degrees of severity. Stress generally makes all these conditions worse.

irritable bowel syndrome (IBS)

This disorder of the lower bowel usually occurs between 20-40 years of age. The usual symptoms are colicky pains, diarrhoea and/or constipation, and distension of the abdomen, giving rise to noisy rumblings and wind. Emotional factors can play an important part in this disorder, and those who are anxious and over-conscientious are the most likely sufferers. Symptoms can be worse just before a period, especially if PMS is present.

It is useful to experiment with diet. Exclude cow's milk and its products and monitor the result. Foods which contain wheat can also cause problems, as can the caffeine in tea and coffee. Try essential oils which balance the digestive system, used in a variety of ways: by ingestion (*see* Aromatherapy Techniques), by application of oils in a carrier base, rubbed on to the abdomen twice daily in a clockwise direction, and by compresses placed over the abdomen.

◁ **The heady yet gentle aroma of rose is a favourite with almost every woman. Rose helps to lift the spirits and promote feelings of well-being.**

cystitis

This is a common problem that can occur after sex and during pregnancy. Cystitis is an infection and inflammation of the bladder and urethra. It is characterized by a frequent, painful urge to go to the toilet. Treatment is with antibacterial and antiseptic essential oils which have an affinity to the kidneys. Cystitis has been treated successfully using a tea with the relevant essential oils added (*see* Aromatherapy Techniques) and by application of the same oils in a carrier base to the abdomen and lower back.

sinusitis

Inflammation of the sinus area around the nose and/or eyes can occur at any time in life after puberty and is often difficult to cure, even with an operation. It causes chronic congestion, catarrh and sometimes headaches. Fortunately, sinusitis can be helped easily and successfully by adding the appropriate essential oils to your regular moisturizer. Allergic reactions or colds can exacerbate the condition, in which case neat essential oils should be inhaled on a tissue or used in the bath. Pressing on the sinus-pressure points on the feet (*see* Swiss Reflex Therapy) every night while symptoms persist is also helpful.

vaginitis

Inflammation of the vagina, with accompanying irritation, can be caused by leaving a tampon in too long or through use of the contraceptive pill. The most frequent cause is when a yeast-like substance, called *Candida albicans*, a normal inhabitant of the mouth and bowel (and, in women, of the vagina) becomes infected. When symptoms first appear, immediate treatment with essential oils will help. Provided a tampon was not the cause of the inflammation in the first place, try a tampon with 2 drops of tea tree oil inserted into the vagina and left in

▷ **An application of fennel, peppermint and/or rosemary can be helpful with IBS. Use in a carrier oil or compress applied to the abdomen area.**

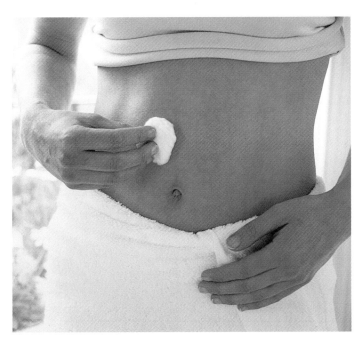

overnight. Alternatively, taking regular sitz-baths for ten minutes at a time, using a synergistic mix of appropriate essential oils, can also help.

thrush

Infected *Candida albicans* can show as white ulcerous spots inside the mouth (thrush), which can be dealt with using a mouthwash including anti-infectious essential oils. The vagina can also be affected with thrush, giving rise to itching and discomfort. Thrush usually affects women with a low immune system, where it can be due to stress, the overuse of antibiotics or diabetes. Additional symptoms which can present themselves at this time include cystitis, depression and headaches.

With thrush it is helpful if the intake of sugar and refined carbohydrates in the diet is reduced immediately. If the condition worsens, an effective form of aromatherapy treatment involves eating live yogurt containing suitable essential oils: 20 drops of oil to 100 ml (6-7 tbsp) of yogurt and, if possible, inserting some of this mixture into the vagina with a tampon applicator.

endometriosis

This condition is when tissue similar to that of the lining of the uterus is found elsewhere – mostly in the ovaries. The tissue swells and bleeds, causing severe pain before a period and excessive blood loss during it. Conventional treatment may recommend removal of the ovaries (and therefore the

△ Peppermint is useful for relieving nasal congestion and treating general sinus problems.

hormone production) so that the uterus is no longer stimulated to produce the extra tissue. The contraceptive pill is often prescribed but this is not always successful.

Some women prefer to avoid surgery if possible, in which case it is worth trying hormone-like and decongestant essential oils first, as they have been known to help. If surgery is inevitable, then oestrogen-like essential oils will help the body to readjust itself to the loss of the ovaries.

◁ A compress of clary sage and cypress can be used for problems associated with the ovaries.

Useful essential oils

essential oil	treatment
stress	
Chamomile (Roman) *Chamaemelum nobile*	calming
Lemon *Citrus limon*	calming, hypotensive
Melissa *Melissa officinalis*	calming, sedative
Ylang ylang *Cananga odorata*	balancing, calming, hypotensive
depression	
Basil *Ocimum basilicum* var. *album*	neurotonic
Frankincense *Boswellia carteri*	energizing, immunostimulant
Juniper *Juniperus communis*	neurotonic
Neroli *Citrus aurantium* var. *amara*	tranquilizing (nervous depression, fatigue)
Niaouli *Melaleuca viridiflora*	tonic
Peppermint *Mentha* x *piperita*	neurotonic
Pine *Pinus sylvestris*	neurotonic
Rosemary *Rosmarinus officinalis*	neurotonic, sexual tonic
stress with depression	
Bergamot *Citrus bergamia*	balancing, calming, sedative, tonic to central nervous system
Clary sage *Salvia sclarea*	balancing, relaxing, neurotonic
Cypress *Cupressus sempervirens*	balancing, calming, neurotonic
Geranium *Pelargonium graveolens*	balancing, relaxing, stimulant (nervous fatigue)
Lavender *Lavandula angustifolia*	balancing, calming, sedative, tonic
Marjoram *Origanum majorana*	balancing, calming, neurotonic
Rose otto *Rosa damascena*	balancing, relaxing, neurotonic, sexual tonic
poor concentration	
Basil *Ocimum basilicum* var. *album*	neurotonic
Bergamot *Citrus bergamia*	balancing, tonic
Thyme (sweet) *Thymus vulgaris*	cardiotonic, neurotonic, immunostimulant
irritable bowel syndrome	
Fennel *Foeniculum vulgare*	analgesic, antispasmodic, digestive (constipation, diarrhoea, flatulence)
Peppermint *Mentha* x *piperita*	analgesic, anti-inflammatory, digestive (diarrhoea, flatulence)
Rosemary *Rosmarinus officinalis*	analgesic, antispasmodic, digestive (constipation, flatulence)

essential oil	treatment
thrush (*Candida albicans*) and vaginitis	
Lavender *Lavandula angustifolia*	analgesic, antifungal, anti-inflammatory
Pine *Pinus sylvestris*	analgesic, antifungal, anti-infectious, anti-inflammatory, neurotonic
Tea tree *Melaleuca alternifolia*	analgesic, antifungal, anti-infectious, anti-inflammatory, immunostimulant, neurotonic
Thyme (sweet) *Thymus vulgaris*	antifungal, anti-infectious, anti-inflammatory, immunostimulant, neurotonic
cystitis	
Eucalyptus *Eucalyptus smithii*	anti-infectious, antiseptic
Juniper *Juniperus communis*	anti-inflammatory, antiseptic
Lavender *Lavandula angustifolia*	anti-inflammatory, antiseptic
Thyme (sweet) *Thymus vulgaris*	anti-infectious, anti-inflammatory, antiseptic
sinusitis	
Eucalyptus *Eucalyptus smithii*	anti-inflammatory, antiseptic
Lavender *Lavandula angustifolia*	anti-inflammatory, anti-infectious, antiseptic
Peppermint *Mentha* x *piperita*	anti-inflammatory, anti-infectious
endometriosis	
Clary sage *Salvia sclarea*	decongestant, oestrogen-like, phlebotonic
Cypress *Cupressus sempervirens*	astringent, hormone-like (ovary problems), phlebotonic
Geranium *Pelargonium graveolens*	analgesic, astringent, cicatrizant, decongestant, phlebotonic, styptic
Rose otto *Rosa damascena*	astringent, cicatrizant, neurotonic, styptic

Sweet scents are the swift vehicles

of still sweeter thoughts.

Walter Savage Landor, 1775–1864.

essential oil	treatment

anger, fear and jealousy

The following essential oils given can benefit all of these emotions. The properties required for each condition are listed first, the oils which follow show the properties each possesses relevant to that particular emotion.

ANGER

essential oil	treatment
Look for oils which are	analgesic, anticatarrhal, anti-inflammatory, antispasmodic, calming, carminative (relieving flatulence), cicatrizant, sedative
Basil *Ocimum basilicum* var. *album*	analgesic, anti-inflammatory, carminative, calming to the nervous system
Bergamot *Citrus bergamia*	antispasmodic, calming, cicatrizant
Geranium *Pelargonium graveolens*	analgesic, anti-inflammatory, antispasmodic, cicatrizant, relaxant
Juniper *Juniperus communis*	analgesic, anticatarrhal, anti-inflammatory
Lavender *Lavandula angustifolia*	analgesic, anti-inflammatory, antispasmodic, calming and sedative, cicatrizant
Lemon *Citrus limon*	anti-inflammatory, antispasmodic, calming, carminative

FEAR

essential oil	treatment
Look for oils which are	antispasmodic, cardiotonic, calming and soothing, digestive, hypotensive, mental stimulant, nausea relief, nerve tonic, respiratory tonic, sedative
Basil *Ocimum basilicum* var. *album*	antispasmodic, cardiotonic, neurotonic
Bergamot *Citrus bergamia*	antispasmodic (indigestion), calming, sedative (agitation), nerve tonic
Geranium *Pelargonium graveolens*	antispasmodic, relaxant
Juniper *Juniperus communis*	digestive tonic, nerve tonic
Lavender *Lavandula angustifolia*	antispasmodic, calming, cardiotonic, hypotensive, sedative
Lemon *Citrus limon*	antispasmodic (diarrhoea normalizing), calming, hypotensive, nausea relief

The flowers anew, returning seasons bring

But beauty faded has no second spring.

From The First Pastoral, Ambrose Philips, 1675–1749.

essential oil	treatment

JEALOUSY

essential oil	treatment
Look for oils which are	antibacterial, antifungal, antiviral, cicatrizant, detoxifying, litholytic
Basil *Ocimum basilicum* var. *album*	antibacterial, antiviral, decongestant (uterine)
Bergamot *Citrus bergamia*	antibacterial, antiviral, cicatrizant
Geranium *Pelargonium graveolens*	antibacterial, antifungal, cicatrizant, decongestant (lymph)
Juniper *Juniperus communis*	detoxifying, litholytic
Lavender *Lavandula angustifolia*	antibacterial, antifungal, cicatrizant
Lemon *Citrus limon*	antibacterial, antifungal, antiviral, litholytic

irritability

essential oil	treatment
Chamomile (Roman) *Chamaemelum nobile*	calming
Cypress *Cupressus sempervirens*	calming
Rose otto *Rosa damascena*	calming

lack of confidence

essential oil	treatment
Basil *Ocimum basilicum* var. *album*	neurotonic
Bergamot *Citrus bergamia*	balancing, tonic to central nervous system
Lavender *Lavandula angustifolia*	balancing, tonic
Marjoram *Origanum majorana*	balancing, neurotonic
Rosemary *Rosmarinus officinalis*	neurotonic
Thyme (sweet) *Thymus vulgaris*	cardiotonic, neurotonic, immunostimulant

The Reproductive Years

The gentle, calming effects of essential oils lend themselves perfectly to alleviating the physical discomforts of menstruation and pregnancy. Aromatic baths, soothing compresses and relaxing massage treatments can all help a woman stay naturally healthy throughout her reproductive years.

Coping with menstruation

When a girl reaches puberty, her previously dormant ovaries begin to release eggs for potential fertilization in the uterus. The ovaries take it in turns, approximately once a month, to release one, or sometimes two, eggs. The length of this cycle varies between individuals, from three to five weeks on average. The menstrual cycle is controlled by several hormones released by the endocrine system: these include oestrogen and progesterone, the latter being responsible for the thickening of the uterus lining, ready to welcome and feed a fertilized egg. At the same time, the breasts begin to swell a little, as they prepare to produce milk-forming tissue, and congestion occurs, particularly in the area between the nipples and the armpits.

If the egg is not fertilized within a few days, it dies and, together with the lining of the uterus, is rejected by the uterus two weeks after its arrival. The result is a flow of blood lasting, on average, between three and five days. Once finished, it can take up to three weeks before the next egg is released, depending on the individual.

This hormonal activity can cause period pain (dysmenorrhoea), irregularity, a heavy blood flow (menorrhagia), hardly

▷ **For some women, their periods are marked by a dull backache. Sweet marjoram, rosemary and pine can be applied on a warm compress to the painful area.**

△ **Peppermint is useful for treating nausea and headaches. It can be taken internally in water.**

any flow (oligomenorrhoea) or perhaps no flow at all (amenorrhoea). Other symptoms may appear, and can vary from water retention, constipation, backache, tiredness, nausea, headaches and migraine, to tender breasts and premenstrual syndrome (PMS). This emotional complication of PMS can adversely affect the rest of the family as well as the sufferer. PMS should not be confused with period pains or any of the other symptoms experienced during menstruation, as the moment blood flow begins, PMS symptoms disappear.

painful periods

These are caused by congestion of blood in the uterus. Symptoms can range from a slight discomfort to a heavy, dragging pain in the abdomen. For some women, period pains may also affect the lower back.

treatment

Apply analgesic and decongestant essential oils in a vegetable oil or lotion carrier-base, in a clockwise direction, over the entire abdomen, daily at bedtime, eight to ten days before your period is due. When you have pain or tender breasts it is beneficial to apply a warm compress, using the same essential oils as above (*see* Aromatherapy Techniques). Exercise can be helpful as it stimulates the blood circulation and relieves congestion. After childbirth, period pains usually diminish or disappear.

irregular, infrequent or lack of periods

This can be very frustrating from the point of view of planning your life, especially if you are trying to conceive a child. The problem is due to hormonal imbalance. Worry can make things worse, so stress-relieving essential oils, when used regularly, can be beneficial.

treatment

Roman chamomile, melissa and rose otto essential oils can be blended together in a carrier-base oil or lotion and rubbed into the abdomen, in a clockwise direction. The appropriate, hormone-like, essential oils should also be used.

LIFESTYLE TIPS FOR MENSTRUAL PROBLEMS

- Foods to avoid: excess sugar, salt, chocolate
- Foods to eat: liver, fish, fresh fruit (especially bananas), nuts, pulses, raw or cooked fresh vegetables (especially greens), salads (with evening primrose oil), diuretic vegetables, such as fennel, cucumber and cabbage (try cooking cabbage in a minimum amount of water and drink the water that is left after cooking).
- Drinks to avoid: excess caffeine found in tea, coffee and cola.

scanty and heavy periods

These may be due to an imbalance of prostaglandin in the body, a hormone which affects the uterus. With heavy periods, the lining of the uterus is over-thick.

treatment

Use hormone-like essential oils.

other symptoms

Constipation, tiredness and backache can all arise as a result of period problems. Other

◁ **Include plenty of fresh fruit in your daily diet. Healthy eating can alleviate period problems.**

△ **Rosemary is a good choice to help with period problems, relieving constipation and fatigue.**

symptoms which can arise around the time of menstruation are associated with PMS.

treatment

Many oils are effective against backache, and it is probably best to experiment until you find the ones you like best. Rosemary and mandarin, used together, are known to be effective for constipation.

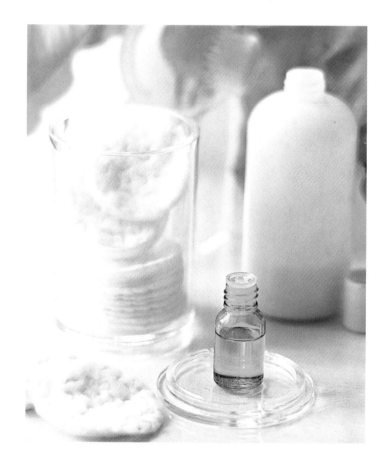

▷ **Experiment with making your own lotions. Choose the oils most suited to your symptoms and have a bottle made up and ready to use.**

Pre-menstrual syndrome (PMS)

Some researchers estimate that PMS affects up to half of adult women living in modern society. No one knows exactly the cause of PMS, but it is believed that the lowered hormone level in the body after the egg has been released is mainly responsible for the collection of mental and physical symptoms which can become apparent eight to ten days before menstruation. Contributory factors include poor nutrition and stress: women often juggle many responsibilities at the same time, with insufficient time to eat properly and relax.

excessive water retention

Fluid retention is thought to be a crucial factor in PMS, as it affects all the cells in the body. PMS may be accompanied by weight gain and shows itself in the swelling of the abdomen, ankles and breasts, which can become very tender and swollen.

treatment

Diuretic and decongestant essential oils can be used to help reduce swelling.

persistent headaches and sleep disturbances

Both a lack of sleep and regular headaches are draining on the body, and will increase stress levels and the inability to cope.

treatment

Calming, neurotonic and decongestant essential oils can be used to relieve the headaches and/or insomnia by balancing the whole body.

emotional instability

Many women suffer from depression and irritability every month. In some cases, this can be severe and can lead to arguments and difficulties at home and at work.

treatment

Antidepressive and calming essential oils, taken as inhalations and baths, can help.

◁ To make a compress, add a few drops of your chosen oil blend to a bowl of water and mix well. Place a piece of cloth on the water's surface and let the oil soak into it. Use as needed.

▽ For sleepless nights, headaches, and irritability prepare a mix of Roman chamomile, melissa and lavender. It may be handy to keep some by your bedside.

LIFESTYLE TIPS FOR PMS

For the most effective results, a holistic approach to PMS is essential.

- Amend your diet to boost your general health and vitality
- Exercise to stimulate your blood circulation and to relieve congestion: try walking, cycling and swimming.
- Avoid stressful situations wherever possible, and ask for help if home or work responsibilities become too much
- Take your favourite relevant essential oils to work for instant therapy

hormonal treatment

Some essential oils have a tendency to normalize hormonal secretions, including those involved in the reproductive system. Cypress is helpful for all ovarian problems. Clary sage and niaouli are oestrogen-like, which makes them useful for the stages in a woman's life when oestrogen production is unstable. To balance your hormones, these oils should be used in applications, baths and inhalations ten to 12 days before the expected start of a period.

Useful essential oils

essential oil	treatment

hormone-like essential oils

essential oil	treatment
Chamomile (German) *Matricaria recutica*	decongestant, hormone-like
Clary sage *Salvia sclarea*	decongestant, oestrogen-like
Cypress *Cupressus sempervirens*	hormone-like (ovarian)
Niaouli *Melaleuca viridiflora*	oestrogen-like (regularizes menses)
Peppermint *Mentha* x *piperita*	hormone-like (ovarian stimulant), neurotonic

painful periods and backache

essential oil	treatment
Basil *Ocimum basilicum* var. *album*	analgesic, antispasmodic, decongestant
Eucalyptus *Eucalyptus smithii* (not *Eucalyptus globulus*)	analgesic, decongestant
Geranium *Pelargonium graveolens*	analgesic, antispasmodic, decongestant
Lavender *Lavandula angustifolia*	analgesic, antispasmodic, calming, sedative, tonic
Marjoram (sweet) *Origanum majorana*	analgesic, antispasmodic, calming, neurotonic
Peppermint *Mentha* x *piperita*	analgesic, decongestant, hormone-like (ovarian stimulant)
Pine *Pinus sylvestris*	analgesic, decongestant
Rosemary *Rosmarinus officinalis*	analgesic, antispasmodic, decongestant

irregular, scanty and/or lack of periods

Mix a blend using the hormone-like essential oils (above).
Other possibilities include:

essential oil	treatment
Chamomile (Roman) *Chamaemelum nobile*	calming, menstrual regulator, nervous menstrual problems
Melissa *Melissa officinalis*	calming, sedative, regularizes secretions
Rose otto *Rosa damascena*	general reproductive system regulator

heavy periods

essential oil	treatment
Cypress *Cupressus sempervirens*	astringent, phlebotonic, hormone-like (ovary problems)
Melissa *Melissa officinalis*	calming, sedative, regularizes secretions

fluid retention

essential oil	treatment
Cypress *Cupressus sempervirens*	diuretic (oedema, rheumatic swelling)
Fennel *Foeniculum vulgare*	diuretic (cellulite, oedema)
Juniper *Juniperus communis*	diuretic (cellulite, oedema)
Sage *Salvia officinalis*	decongestant, lypolytic (cellulite)

low spirits (depression) and fatigue

essential oil	treatment
Basil *Ocimum basilicum* var. *album*	nervous system regulator (anxiety), neurotonic (convalescence, depression)
Chamomile (Roman) *Chamaemelum nobile*	calming (nervous depression, nervous shock)
Clary sage *Salvia sclarea*	neurotonic (nervous fatigue)
Geranium *Pelargonium graveolens*	relaxant (anxiety, debility, nervous fatigue)
Juniper *Juniperus communis*	neurotonic (debility, fatigue)
Marjoram (sweet) *Origanum majorana*	neurotonic (debility, mental instability, anguish, nervous depression)
Pine *Pinus sylvestris*	neurotonic (debility, fatigue)
Rosemary *Rosmarinus officinalis*	neurotonic (general debility and fatigue)

tender, congested breasts

essential oil	treatment
Eucalyptus *Eucalyptus smithii* (not *Eucalyptus globulus*)	analgesic, decongestant
Geranium *Pelargonium graveolens*	analgesic, decongestant

headaches

essential oil	treatment
Chamomile (Roman) *Chamaemelum nobile*	antispasmodic, calming, sedative
Lavender *Lavandula angustifolia*	analgesic, calming, sedative
Marjoram (sweet) *Origanum majorana*	analgesic, antispasmodic, calming
Melissa *Melissa officinalis*	calming, sedative
Peppermint *Mentha* x *piperita*	analgesic, antispasmodic
Rosemary *Rosmarinus officinalis*	analgesic, antispasmodic, decongestant

insomnia

essential oil	treatment
Basil *Ocimum basilicum* var. *album*	nervous system regulator (nervous insomnia)
Chamomile (Roman) *Chamaemelum nobile*	calming, sedative
Lavender *Lavandula angustifolia*	calming, sedative
Lemon *Citrus limon*	calming
Melissa *Melissa officinalis*	calming, sedative

irritability

essential oil	treatment
Chamomile (Roman) *Chamaemelum nobile*	calming, sedative

Preparing for pregnancy

Once the menstrual cycle begins, becoming pregnant is a possibility until periods end at the menopause. Once an egg is fertilized, the body's hormones begin to change and can give rise to many symptoms, some of which can be helped with essential oils.

after conception

A normal pregnancy lasts approximately nine months. It is divided into three periods of approximately three months, known as trimesters. Once you realize that you are pregnant, you may experience a variety of emotions, ranging from joy and delight to fear and apprehension. Towards the end of the first trimester your breasts may feel tender and your appetite may increase. At this stage you may develop a heightened sense of smell, and this may start to affect your food preferences.

The second trimester is probably the most enjoyable, as you gradually become accustomed to the physical and emotional aspects of having a baby. During this time, you can benefit from using essential oils to help with some of the stresses and strains you may be experiencing as you adjust to

the changes that are taking place in your body. Remember that any essential oils you use for yourself will also reach your baby, and they should be used with care and common sense if you are both to reap the benefits.

By the third trimester you will look well and truly pregnant and your body will start to feel heavy and cumbersome. During this time you need more rest, preferably with your feet up, and you will be starting to make preparations for labour.

Throughout the pregnancy be sure to eat well. You also need to look after your teeth: your baby will take from you whatever nutrition he or she needs and it is you who will be deprived of essential nutrients such as calcium and iron. Listen to your body: a food craving can often indicate your baby's and your own body's needs. For example, a craving for cheese could mean your body needs more calcium and protein.

cautions during pregnancy

You may not know you are pregnant until two months have already passed. If you are trying to conceive, you should use only the

△ **Fresh flowers bring beauty into our lives and stimulate feelings of happiness and well-being.**

more popular essential oils, in general use, at this time. By the fifth month of pregnancy, the baby should be firmly attached to the uterus, and any essential oils can be used. All essential oils should be used only in the recommended dosage.

Some essential oils have components in them which may induce a period or which can affect the nervous system if overused. Some of these oils may help to stimulate the uterus into action, and they should be used only when labour commences, to relieve labour pains. Used correctly, essential oils can alleviate many of the minor discomforts of pregnancy. Many women also find them invaluable during labour to ease pain and to facilitate delivery. However, some controversy exists surrounding the use of some essential oils during pregnancy.

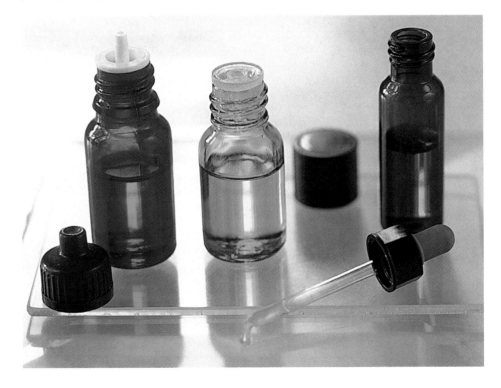

◁ **Two essential oils can be mixed together in an easy-to-use dropper bottle for effective self-treatment at home.**

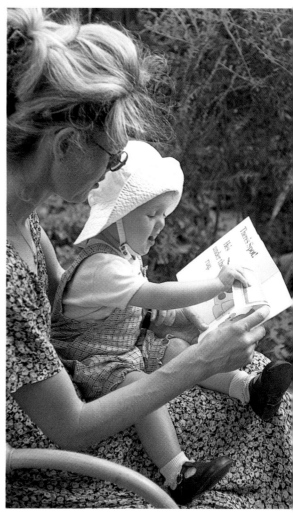

◁ A cool lavender compress can ease a tension headache. Lie or sit quietly in a place where you won't be disturbed and apply the compress to your temples or forehead until relief is felt.

▽ Whether this is your first pregnancy or whether you are already a mother, preparing for a new baby is an exciting time for all the family.

A few essential oils have the ability to stimulate uterine contractions, and could possibly cause miscarriage if taken in excessive amounts or taken internally during the first three to four months of pregnancy. Other oils can have an effect on the nervous system and the liver, and could be toxic when taken in too high a dose.

When oils are used correctly, the risks are very slight because of the low dosage involved (generally, five to ten drops at any one time). Women who have a history of miscarriage may be most at risk but, in any case, it is always better to err on the side of safety. Use only those essential oils which do not appear in any literature as being hazardous during pregnancy. There are many oils which will do you no harm at all but, if you are in any doubt about using an essential oil while pregnant, you should consult a qualified aromatherapist.

Whether pregnant or trying to start a family, the important thing to remember is that anything taken into the body, whether it is food, drink, nicotine, alcohol, or any other substance, will have an effect upon the system. Sensible eating with plenty of sleep and regular exercise is the best way to look after yourself and prepare your body and mind for motherhood.

OILS TO AVOID DURING THE FIRST HALF OF PREGNANCY

Although all essential oils are safe when used with care and knowledge, it is advised that you avoid the following oils, which can promote menstruation:

- aniseed *Pimpinella anisum*
- fennel *Foeniculum vulgare*
- nutmeg *Myristica fragrans*
- sage *Salvia officinalis*
- yarrow *Achillea millefolium*

In addition, avoid any essential oil that is new to you at this time.

Using aromatherapy in pregnancy

Essential oils can bring relief from the many minor troubles which can occur during pregnancy. Discomforts commonly experienced by women include morning sickness, backache, oedema (swollen legs and ankles), constipation, varicose veins, digestive problems (including heartburn), leg cramps and exhaustion. Coping with these discomforts can be especially difficult while the woman is working or if there is a small child or children to look after in the home. Essential oils are also useful during labour, to ease pain and to facilitate delivery.

morning sickness

Nausea, which typically occurs in the morning, is often one of the first signs that a woman is pregnant. Inhalations with a vaporizer can be helpful at bedtime and first thing in the morning. The oils can be left to vaporize overnight in the bedroom. If the sickness persists through the day, prepare a tissue with the relevant oils, and keep it with you at all times.

constipation

This is also another early sign of pregnancy. Prepare essential oils in a suitable carrier base and apply them to the abdomen in a

△ **As your pregnancy proceeds, you will feel your baby's first movements. Setting aside some time each day to relax and be with your unborn child can help the mother-child bonding process.**

◁ **Add a few drops of bitter orange to a bowl of water and make a compress to ease constipation.**

clockwise direction. Alternatively, use the oils in the bath and/or on a compress. Eating a healthy diet and drinking plenty of water will help to reduce the risk of constipation.

stretch marks

By the beginning of the second trimester, your clothes will be feeling tighter as your abdomen swells. Halfway through this trimester you will be able to feel the baby's first movements (an exciting moment). Start using essential oils at this time to prevent stretch marks on the skin of the abdomen. Through the correct and diligent

application of appropriate essential oils it is possible to maintain a supple and undamaged skin, and you will greatly appreciate your efforts after the baby is born.

Prepare a carrier base (include calendula oil) containing oils with regenerative and skin-toning properties. The mixture should be applied to the abdomen twice daily, morning and night. The area to be covered increases as the pregnancy proceeds, and will include the sides of the body, the groin and on and above the breasts.

backache

As your baby grows, so the likelihood of backache increases. Sitting and standing with correct posture can go a long way to minimize backache, but it will usually occur at some stage and can be helped with essential oils when it does. Prepare a carrier base, then add the appropriate oils and ask a friend or your partner to give you a back massage, ideally at bedtime. Try using the same essential oils (but without the carrier oil) in the bath. Include basil and marjoram in the massage-mix; these can also be used if you suffer from leg cramps later on.

heartburn

The growing baby may also put pressure on your stomach, causing indigestion and heartburn. For heartburn, add 2 drops each of mandarin and peppermint oils to 10 ml (2 tsp) carrier base and apply to the painful area. These oils can also be inhaled neat from a tissue or cupped hands, breathing deeply.

varicose veins, swollen legs and ankles

It is as well for all women to watch out for early signs of these conditions throughout pregnancy. Resting with the feet and legs raised is beneficial for all leg conditions. Although the essential oils are different for each condition, the method of use is the same. Prepare a carrier base and add the oils.

◁ Your growing baby can cause painful heartburn. Put two drops each of mandarin and peppermint on a tissue and sniff throughout the day.

▽ Backache is a common complaint of pregnancy. Ask your partner for a back massage, using basil and marjoram, before going to bed.

Apply the mixture to the whole leg, then bring your hands firmly from the foot up to the knee, before returning to the foot to start again. Massage only in an upward direction, to encourage blood flow to the heart. For varicose veins on the upper leg, massage upwards, going only from knee to groin – not back again – several times.

◁ A room vaporizer is a convenient way of inhaling oils. To help with morning sickness, vaporize a combination of lemon, ginger and basil at bedtime and when you wake up.

Ante-natal bodycare

During the last trimester of pregnancy, it is a good idea to prepare for labour and to discuss with your midwife or doctor how you would like the birth to proceed. It is helpful to attend prenatal classes, especially if it is the birth of your first child. The classes teach useful exercises to help you relax when the time for labour comes.

preparing for labour

Much of the pain of childbirth, particularly with a first child, is due to the muscles at the neck of the uterus and the perineum being tense and/or inflexible, which means they can tear when stretched. This can be eased by the application of muscle-relaxing essential oils in a vegetable carrier oil. If application is begun daily from several weeks before the expected birth date, the area can be made supple and soft. This will prepare it for the enormous amount of expansion needed for the baby to be born.

Massage a little of the mix twice daily around the perineum area, and try inserting your fingers into the neck of the womb to stretch it, thus helping to prevent tearing.

◁ **To prevent stretch marks, geranium and frankincense, in a calendula oil carrier, should be massaged on to the abdomen area twice daily.**

▽ **Massage the lower leg in an upwards direction to relieve aches and oedema.**

As you get heavier, remember to keep increasing the area to which you are applying your essential oil blend to prevent stretch marks, taking your mix round the sides of your body, on to the upper part of your thighs and above your breasts. It is also important at this time to rest your legs at regular intervals (from every five minutes to half an hour, if you suspect you are likely to develop varicose veins).

As the time for the birth approaches, you may experience conflicting emotions and mood swings. Using uplifting essential oils can give you inner strength to cope with all that is in store for you during this very exciting time in your life.

◁ **Make regular checks for oedema on your feet and ankles as your pregnancy progresses. If symptoms occur, a massage plan can help.**

Relief treatments for labour

There are some oils which are particularly useful in labour. In the past, these were limited to lavender and clary sage for their calming and relaxing effects. However, there are a few oils with womb-stimulant and analgesic properties, and these can help with contractions: aniseed, clove bud, nutmeg and sage. These oils are *absolutely not* advocated for the first four months of pregnancy and should not be used until the last week, when labour is about to begin. Used correctly, these oils can help to make the birth easier and quicker, especially for a first-time mother. They are used to relieve pain and induce sleep, and will have a soothing, dulling, lulling effect. Clove bud is particularly analgesic and nutmeg is an effective sedative.

treatment

Try a mix of two drops each of any two of the oils with four drops of lavender on a tissue, and inhale between contractions. Some women like to put the tissue into the switched-off gas and air machine, which seems to have the psychological effect of making the oils more efficient.

Alternatively, blend three drops each of aniseed, nutmeg and peppermint with eight drops of lavender into 50 ml (2 fl oz) carrier oil, and ask your partner to massage your feet and lower legs every half hour. Apply the same mix to your own hands and shoulders, if preferred.

▷ **Lower back pain can be eased by massage. Ask your partner to rub the painful areas.**

◁ **Peppermint and aniseed are analgesic and antispasmodic. Combined with lavender, a blend can be massaged on to the lower legs during labour to ease pain.**

▷ **Inhalation is the fastest method for an oil's aroma to reach the brain. Aniseed and lavender are calming and can help with contractions.**

▷ **Nutmeg is a very useful oil for the last stages of labour as it relieves pain and can facilitate delivery. Consult a qualified aromatherapist if you wish to use it.**

Post-natal bodycare

Essential oils can be used to help with the common emotional stresses and physical problems arising as a result of the birth.

Use 6 drops of the appropriate essential oils blended in 20 ml (4 tsp) of calendula oil for application. Alternatively, use them on their own for inhalation or in the bath.

birth wounds

During the birth, the perineum may be bruised and/or torn, and can be very painful afterwards. Using the three perineum oils, gently apply them several times a day. If the area is too painful to touch, use a compress (*see* Aromatherapy Techniques).

breast feeding problems

Always apply the appropriate essential oils immediately after each feed, so that they are completely absorbed by your body before the baby's next feed is due.

Insufficient milk: fennel oil encourages milk production. Fennel will also help to keep the baby's excreta normal and can help to relieve any wind.
Too much milk: 2 drops of peppermint oil with 4 drops of geranium oil can be used in a massage all over the breasts.
Cracked nipples or mastitis: use 2 drops of each essential oil listed opposite.

emotional difficulties

After the birth, it will take a while before your hormones return to normal. This can be a stressful time as you have a new baby to care for just when you are feeling in need of care yourself. Fatigue, anxiety, despondency and emotional imbalances are common. Essential oils can help before post-natal depression sets in. Blend oils for use by inhalation, in the bath or by application.

treating your baby

Essential oils can help you and your baby cope with the everyday, minor ailments which many babies are subject to, such as

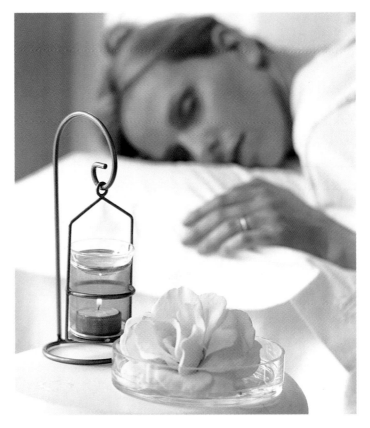

◁ **After a long and exhausting labour, and with a new baby to look after, make sure you get enough sleep. Burn lavender through the night to relax and refresh you.**

▽ **Once your baby is born, pamper yourself and invest in some good quality skincare products.**

△ **The gentle action of mandarin makes it a good choice for treating colic and digestive disorders.**

indigestion, colic, constipation and/or diarrhoea, minor infections and nappy rash. For nappy rash, use 15 ml (3 tsp) base lotion with 5 ml (1 tsp) calendula oil, mixed with one drop of peppermint and up to three drops of any other selected oils.

Babies can benefit from massage with essential oils. The massage will relax them and can help to strengthen the bond between mother and child. For application to babies, use one drop of essential oil per 5 ml (1 tsp) carrier lotion or oil. For sleep problems, try two to three drops of oil in a vaporizer in the baby's room, or try them on a tissue which is pinned to the baby's clothes or placed inside the pillowcase.

Useful essential oils

essential oil	treatment
hormone-like essential oils	
Chamomile (German) *Matricaria recutica*	hormone-like
Clary sage *Salvia sclarea*	oestrogen-like
Niaouli *Melaleuca viridiflora*	oestrogen-like (regularizes periods)
backache	
Basil *Ocimum basilicum* var. *album*	analgesic, antispasmodic
Lavender *Lavandula angustifolia*	analgesic, anti-inflammatory, antispasmodic
Marjoram (sweet) *Origanum majorana*	analgesic, antispasmodic
constipation	
Ginger *Zingiber officinale*	analgesic, digestive stimulant
Mandarin *Citrus reticulata*	antispasmodic, calming, digestive stimulant
Orange (bitter) *Citrus aurantium* var. *amara*	calming, digestive stimulant
Rosemary *Rosmarinus officinalis*	analgesic, digestive stimulant
nausea	
Basil *Ocimum basilicum* var. *album*	digestive tonic, nervous system regulator
Ginger *Zingiber officinale*	digestive
Lemon *Citrus limon*	anticoagulant, antispasmodic, calming, digestive
stretch marks	
Frankincense *Boswellia carteri*	cell regenerative, cicatrizant (scars)
Geranium *Pelargonium graveolens*	cell regenerative, cicatrizant (stretch marks)
Lavender *Lavandula angustifolia*	cicatrizant (scars)
fluid retention	
Fennel *Foeniculum vulgare*	diuretic (cellulite, oedema)
Juniper *Juniperus communis*	diuretic (cellulite, oedema)
Lemon *Citrus limon*	diuretic (obesity, oedema)
varicose veins	
Clary sage *Salvia sclarea*	phlebotonic (circulatory problems, haemorrhoids, varicose veins)
Cypress *Cupressus sempervirens*	phlebotonic (haemorrhoids, poor venous circulation, varicose veins)
Niaouli *Melaleuca viridiflora*	phlebotonic (haemorrhoids, varicose veins)

essential oil	treatment
labour	
Aniseed *Pimpinella anisum*	analgesic, antispasmodic, calming (gentle narcotic), emmenagogic, oestrogen-like, uterotonic
Lavender *Lavandula angustifolia*	analgesic, antispasmodic, calming (anxiety), sedative
Nutmeg *Myristica fragrans*	analgesic, sedative (narcotic), neurotonic, uterotonic
Peppermint *Mentha* x *piperita*	analgesic, antispasmodic, hormone-like (ovarian stimulant), neurotonic, uterotonic (facilitates delivery)
perineum	
Geranium *Pelargonium graveolens*	analgesic, cicatrizant (wounds)
Lavender *Lavandula angustifolia*	analgesic, antiseptic (bruises)
Rosemary *Rosmarinus officinalis*	analgesic, anti-inflammatory
breast milk	
Fennel *Foeniculum vulgare*	lactogenic (promotes milk), oestrogen-like (insufficient milk)
Geranium *Pelargonium graveolens*	decongestant (breast congestion – for too much milk)
Peppermint *Mentha* x *piperita*	antilactogenic (prevents milk forming)
cracked nipples or mastitis	
Chamomile (German) *Matricaria recutica*	cicatrizant (infected wounds, ulcers)
Geranium *Pelargonium graveolens*	cicatrizant (burns, cuts, ulcers, wounds)
Lavender *Lavandula angustifolia*	cicatrizant (burns, scars, varicose veins, wounds)
nappy rash	
Patchouli *Pogostemon patchouli*	anti-inflammatory, cicatrizant (cracked skin, scar tissue)
Peppermint *Mentha* x *piperita*	analgesic, anti-inflammatory, soothing (skin irritation, rashes)
post-natal depression	
Basil *Ocimum basilicum* var. *album*	nervous system regulator (anxiety), neurotonic (convalescence, depression)
Chamomile (Roman) *Chamaemelum nobile*	calming (nervous depression, nervous shock)

The Sunset Years

The onset of the menopause can bring with it physical and emotional problems that can be relieved by the use of essential oils. As we continue to age, essential oil treatments can play their part as a safeguard against the onset of more serious concerns of circulatory disorders, arthritis and digestive problems.

The menopause

The word menopause derives from the Greek words for month, *men*, and halt, *pausis*. It refers to the end of menstruation, when a woman's ovaries no longer produce eggs for fertilization and her periods stop. The accepted average age at which the menopause occurs is 51, with around five per cent of women ceasing their periods before they are 45.

The menopause does not happen overnight. It is a gradual process brought about by growing irregularity in, and gradual reduction of, the reproductive hormones, oestrogen and progesterone. Oestrogen is probably the most important hormone concerned with a woman's health: it helps to lower cholesterol levels, protect against heart attacks and strokes, to preserve bone tissue and regulate mood and behaviour patterns. Instability occurs in the mental and physical body because of these reduced hormone levels. The early stages of the menopause can present similar emotional imbalances to PMS, and physical symptoms, to varying degrees of severity, may also develop.

As with menstruation, different women will be affected in different ways by the menopause. For women who have had a lifetime of period-associated problems, the menopause may come as a welcome relief.

△ **The menopause is a major life transition. How we cope with it will depend to some extent on our mental attitude. Staying in touch with friends and leading an active life can help us to feel positive.**

She is clothed with strength and dignity and can laugh at years to come. She speaks with wisdom and faithful instruction is on her tongue.

From Proverbs 31:25 The Holy Bible.

Once a woman's periods have stopped for a year, there is no longer any need to worry about becoming pregnant or, therefore, to practise any form of birth control. Some women experience few or no problems at all with the menopause, yet for others, this can be a difficult time as their bodies adjust to a major life change.

Other physical changes may be noticed, affecting the skin and hair, the activity of the thyroid glands and the distribution of body fat. Some women may experience sudden haemorrhaging, headaches, dizzy spells and sleep disturbances.

osteoporosis

One of the more serious potential side effects of the menopause is the development of osteoporosis, which is caused by lack of oestrogen production. This is when the bones of the body become increasingly fragile and brittle. The bones fracture easily, particularly at the more vulnerable points such as the wrists, ankles or hip joints in the event of physical stress, such as a fall. Osteoporosis is also responsible for the eventual development of stooping shoulders in older women, often referred to as a "dowager's hump".

◁ **With the children grown up, you are likely to have more time for yourself. Now is a good time to catch up with family and friends.**

Hormone replacement therapy

Advances in medical science now mean that synthetic hormone replacements can offset the symptoms of the menopause. Many women decide to try hormone replacement therapy (HRT) if they find that the discomforts of the menopause are affecting their quality of life. HRT is not suitable for all women, however, and much

will depend on the needs and medical background of the individual. Because HRT is still a relatively new treatment, its long-term effects are not yet fully known. Treatments are now available from your doctor which are made with natural progesterone. These are believed to be safer than treatments using synthetic oestrogen, and this will make them popular with many women.

Some menopausal symptoms can also be helped by aromatherapy. Clary sage is one of several oestrogen-like essential oils. It is worth using essential oils on a regular basis to see how your symptoms are affected before deciding on HRT.

▽ **Clary sage and cypress can help with night sweats. Prepare a mix and use it at bedtime.**

COMMON SYMPTOMS OF THE MENOPAUSE
- Hot flushes
- Night sweats
- Depression
- Sweating
- Fatigue
- Water retention
- Vaginal dryness

▷ **Some women choose to spend more time on gardening or other hobbies, while others may decide to retrain and embark on a new career.**

Common symptoms of menopause

Although a large percentage of women have no problems with the menopause, many do experience some discomfort.

night sweats

These are best tackled through preventative treatment. Try taking an aromatherapy bath with the relevant oils each night before bedtime. Alternatively, try massaging the oils in a suitable carrier base into the body.

hot flushes

Put 20 drops of the same blend of essential oils in 1 litre (1¾ pints) of spring water in a screw-topped bottle. Fit the lid, shake well and transfer some into a purse-size spray and some into a small bottle that you can carry around with you. As soon as you feel a flush coming on, drink two mouthfuls of the water and spray your face and neck. Vitamin E is also said to be effective.

water retention and bloating

To reduce water retention and cellulite, the relevant essential oils should be added to a suitable carrier base and applied daily to the affected areas. The same oils can also be used neat in the bath.

△ **Rose otto can help with haemorrhaging. It is also useful for both loss of libido and dry skin.**

hair and skin

The condition of the hair and skin can be affected by the hormonal changes of the menopause. Both will become thinner and drier, and it is a good idea to adapt your daily care regime to compensate.

hair

For hair dryness, use a good conditioner. You may like to add appropriate essential oils to give extra shine. For thinning hair, try a daily scalp massage with essential oils (*see* Aromatherapy Techniques).

skin

This not only becomes drier, but is more prone to wrinkles. Try a product containing essential oils or prepare your own mix.

haemorrhaging

Occasional and sudden bleeding can occur when you least expect it. Although essential oils can reduce the amount of blood loss, as far as we know, they do not seem to stop it happening. As a preventative measure, try using styptic and/or astringent essential oils if you are prone to haemorrhaging.

◁ **Peppermint and cypress are useful for hot flushes. Make up a mix and use it in an atomizer.**

△ A refreshing lemon drink can give you a boost and relieve depression. As always, special care should be taken with oils for internal use.

△ If you are having difficulties sleeping, a soothing cup of sweet marjoram and chamomile tea in the evening can help.

◁ Make your own beauty products by adding combinations of your favourite oils to quality base creams and lotions.

heart and circulation problems

In developed countries, arterial disease is the commonest cause of death for women over 50, killing one in four. This is almost twice as high as the death-rate from cancer.

There are as yet no essential oils known to treat problems with the heart, and it is advisable to check with your doctor and your family history to see if you are at risk. In the meantime, you can help to prevent heart and blood-pressure problems by giving up smoking, avoiding fatty foods and drinks high in caffeine, eating a low-cholesterol diet and taking enough regular exercise. There are also some carrier oils reputed to reduce cholesterol levels.

vaginal dryness

This can cause both emotional and physical discomfort. There are no known essential oils to increase vaginal fluid. Vitamin E is reputed to improve vaginal secretion, and daily application of sunflower oil all round the vaginal opening may also help.

Emotions during menopause

For many women the menopause will coincide with their children leaving home. It can represent a new lease of life as a woman suddenly finds that she has more time for herself. However, as with any major life change, the menopause is often accompanied by mixed feelings, and a woman's new-found freedom may be marred not only by physical symptoms but also by emotional disturbances.

stress-related headaches and sleep disturbances

These disturbances are not necessarily linked to the menopause, and may be stress-related. However, should either of them bother you, inhalation and application of the appropriate essential oils can help.

weight and diet

Appearance is often important to a woman throughout her life. It is not surprising, then, that poor self-esteem and a lack of confidence can be triggered by the physical changes happening in her body at this time.

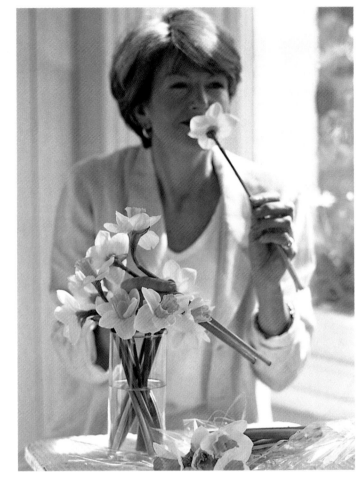

◁ **During the menopause, you may experience strong mood swings. Try to keep things in proportion and take pleasure from the simple things in life.**

△ **When you are feeling tired and irritable, a head massage can help you to relax and unwind.**

Water retention can lead to bloating and weight-gain which, in turn, will exacerbate any feelings of low self-esteem. Tackle this with a positive frame of mind and healthy eating habits – these two things combined will improve self-confidence. Essential oils used for low spirits may help weight loss by stimulating the nervous system.

EMOTIONAL DISTURBANCES OF THE MENOPAUSE

- Irritability
- Lack of confidence
- Anxiety and depression
- Poor concentration, forgetfulness and memory problems
- Decrease in self-esteem: through weight gain, lack of interest in sex, changes in physical appearance

tips for healthy eating and drinking

- Drink plenty of water.
- Limit alcohol intake to two units a day.
- Cut down on caffeine drinks.
- Cut down on, or avoid, sugary foods and foods high in fat.
- Eat more fish and less meat (especially red meat); eat plenty of fruit and vegetables, especially those rich in Vitamin C.
- Include foods rich in calcium.

loss of sex drive

For some women, the menopause is marked by a decrease in sex drive (conversely, some women also report an increase in libido). The reduction in vaginal fluid can make intercourse painful, and this can lead to a change in sexual desire.

Several essential oils are reputed to help with sexual problems and to increase desire. These oils relax the mind, relieving it from pressures and tensions and, at the same time, can stimulate the emotions. Use the appropriate oils in a vaporizer for an hour before retiring, in both the living room and the bedroom. Alternatively, sprinkle a few drops of the oils on to your pillow and exchange a gentle back and shoulder aromatherapy massage with your partner.

relationship difficulties

The physical and emotional difficulties of the menopause can put a strain on your relationship with your partner. If your children are leaving home, now may be a good time to re-define your partnership. It can help to blend stress-relieving essential oils with oils which correspond to your emotions, such as anger, fear or jealousy.

▷ **Emotional upsets are stressful and can lead to muscular tension. Rub oils on to your shoulders and neck to help restore your equilibrium.**

Useful essential oils

essential oil	treatment
hot flushes and sweating	
Clary sage *Salvia sclarea*	antisudorific, oestrogen-like (sweating)
Cypress *Cupressus sempervirens*	antisudorific (excessive perspiration)
Peppermint *Mentha* x *piperita*	cooling
Pine *Pinus sylvestris*	antisudorific (sweating)
reputed sexual stimulants	
Peppermint *Mentha* x *piperita*	neurotonic, reproductive tonic
Rosemary *Rosmarinus officinalis*	neurotonic, sexual tonic
Rose otto *Rosa damascena*	neurotonic, sexual tonic
Thyme (sweet) *Thymus vulgaris*	cardiotonic, immunostimulant, neurotonic, sexual tonic
Ylang ylang *Cananga odorata*	reproductive tonic
low spirits (depression) and fatigue	
Basil *Ocimum basilicum* var. *album*	neurotonic debility, mental strain, depression
Chamomile (Roman) *Chamaemelum nobile*	calming (nervous depression, irritability, nervous shock)
Clary sage *Salvia sclarea*	neurotonic (nervous fatigue)
Cypress *Cupressus sempervirens*	neurotonic (debility)
Frankincense *Boswellia carteri*	antidepressive (nervous depression)
Geranium *Pelargonium graveolens*	neurotonic (debility, nervous fatigue)
Juniper *Juniperus communis*	neurotonic (debility, fatigue)
Marjoram (sweet) *Origanum majorana*	neurotonic (debility, anguish, agitation, nervous depression)
Rosemary *Rosmarinus officinalis*	neurotonic (general debility and fatigue)

essential oil	treatment
fluid retention and cellulite	
Cypress *Cupressus sempervirens*	diuretic (oedema, rheumatic swelling)
Geranium *Pelargonium graveolens*	decongestant (lymphatic congestion)
headaches and sleep problems	
Chamomile (Roman) *Chamaemelum nobile*	antispasmodic, calming (migraines, insomnia, irritability)
Lavender *Lavandula angustifolia*	analgesic, calming (headaches, migraines, insomnia – low dose)
Marjoram (sweet) *Origanum majorana*	analgesic, calming (agitation, migraines, insomnia)
headaches and migraines only	
Peppermint *Mentha* x *piperita*	analgesic (headaches, migraine)
Rosemary *Rosmarinus officinalis*	decongestant (headaches, migraine)
irritability	
Chamomile (Roman) *Chamaemelum nobile*	calming (irritability, nervous depression, nervous shock)
Cypress *Cupressus sempervirens*	calming (irritability), regulates sympathetic nervous system
haemorrhage	
Cypress *Cupressus sempervirens*	astringent, phlebotonic (broken capillaries, varicose veins)
Rose otto *Rosa damascena*	astringent, styptic (wounds)

Aging gracefully

Once the menopause is over women enter a new phase of life, sometimes referred to as "the sunset years", before reaching old-age. During these years it is especially important for women to take care of themselves so as to prolong a happy, healthy and active life.

During the aging process, circulation slows down and the body's cells neither receive nourishment nor have harmful toxins eliminated as quickly as before. As a result, circulatory disorders are common: the hands and feet become cold, and wounds take longer to heal, for example. Digestive disorders in the elderly are also quite common. As the digestive processes slow down and the large intestine muscles weaken, constipation may occur. This is made more likely by inadequate roughage and fibre in the diet, and can also be seen as a side effect of other medicines. Eating while anxious or frightened can also bring on a variety of digestive disorders.

All cell renewal takes longer with age, the skin becomes dry and flaky, and the hair often becomes thinner. Because of this

An essence of balm (melissa) given in Canary wine every morning will renew youth, strengthen the brain, relieve languishing nature and prevent baldness.

From the London Dispensary, 1696.

slowing down process, every organ of every system in the body is more susceptible to common illnesses, which are more difficult to shake off. Older people are particularly vulnerable to colds and 'flu, which can settle on the chest, causing or exacerbating respiratory problems such as bronchitis and asthma. The joints gradually become less

flexible and the muscles are more prone to inflammation, and conditions such as arthritis or rheumatism may develop or get worse. As it is often first highlighted during the menopause, osteoporosis can become a problem, with the skeletal bones becoming more brittle: falls resulting in broken bones, such as the hip, are much more common in later years.

For many women, the prospect of old age is very frightening and creates tension and anxiety. Many women worry about the possibility of incapacitating illnesses, such as dementia, Parkinson's or Alzheimer's disease. Others suffer frequent headaches, migraines, insomnia and digestive upsets, which may be caused by the side effects of medical drugs that are being taken for other conditions. In fact, the side effects of medication can be responsible for many ailments apparent in older people. This can set up a vicious circle, where new medicines are prescribed to deal with the side effects of the original drug and which, in turn, can eventually lead to even more unpleasant

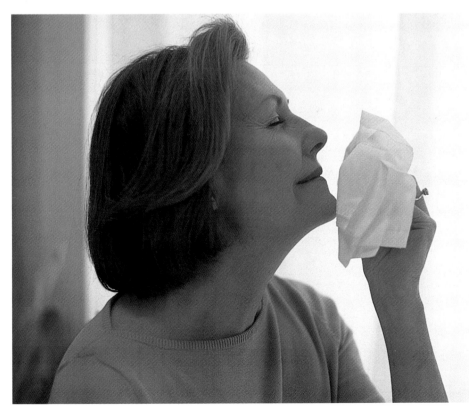

◁ **Extra care should be taken with a cold as it can develop into bronchitis. Use pine and niaouli on a tissue and inhale throughout the day.**

◁ Striking a healthy balance between relaxation and activity is important. Besides keeping you company, a dog will encourage you to take a daily walk.

symptoms. These resulting afflictions are termed iatrogenic because they arise as the side effects of medication taken for the original disease or problem. Aromatherapy is now used in a growing number of hospitals to alleviate the more minor, but unpleasant, effects of iatrogenic disease: insomnia and digestive disorders are the most common, followed by pressure sores for those who are bedridden.

aromatherapy in later life

For women in their later years the amount of essential oils to be used in any treatment depends on the state of their general health. For those in good mental and physical health, the normal number of drops can be used. For women who are run down, suffering ill-health or are on medication the dosage should be lowered, as follows (*see also* Aromatherapy Techniques).

dosage

in the bath 4–6 drops of oil dispersed or dissolved first in dairy cream or honey
for application to the body 8–10 drops in 50 ml (3½ tbsp) carrier lotion
for inhalation the number of drops here is not crucial as many of the molecules are carried away by evaporation.

When preparing oils for application, a lotion is the preferred choice for a carrier base: oil bases can cause bottles to become too slippery and messy, often resulting in oil stains. If you suffer from arthritis, for example, you can add the relevant essential oils to a base hand and/or body lotion, to make the treatment easier to administer.

◁ Holding a cotton pad with a few drops each of sweet marjoram and melissa to your head can relieve a tension headache. If it persists, try adding a few drops of Roman chamomile.

Strengthening physical health

In our sunset years, we have the time to look after our health. Now is the time to use essential oils as a safeguard against problems starting in the first place.

circulatory disorders

The regular daily use of hand and/or body lotion containing the appropriate essential oils will maintain a healthy circulation. Used early enough this could delay and, in some cases, prevent, many circulatory problems occurring.

After a stroke, the daily application of a lotion blend to legs and arms, in an upward direction only (to aid blood flow towards the heart), can help to regain movement in affected limbs.

varicose ulcers

These ulcers can originate from varicose veins, but they can also arise as secondary symptoms of diabetes, sickle-cell anaemia and rheumatoid arthritis. Essential oils dispersed in water and sprayed on to the area is the best method if the ulcers are too raw to touch. A compress is the next step, followed by application with oils in a calendula base as soon as the area can be touched.

arthritis, rheumatism and osteoarthritis

The main symptoms of arthritis are pain and stiffness, and of rheumatoid arthritis, inflammation and swelling around the joints, especially the knuckles, wrists, knees and ankles. Osteoarthritis is degeneration of the joint cartilage. A common site is the hip and, often, the only cure is to have an artificial hip replacement. Aromatherapy helps to alleviate pain and improve mobility in arthritic joints. The recommended treatment is the twice-daily use of a lotion containing relevant essential oils gently massaged into the affected knees or hips. Use overnight compresses for affected hands and feet.

△ **Gentle exercise helps to keep arthritis at bay and maintain a healthy circulatory system**.

bronchial asthma and bronchitis

Many of the expectorant essential oils, which ease breathing, come from the conifer and melaleuca families, such as pine and niaouli. Try application of the oils in a carrier lotion, rubbed into the chest at bedtime. If a visit to hospital is necessary for any reason, take the lotion with you as it will help to prevent infections, such as pneumonia, which are often picked up in hospital.

influenza

Many essential oils are anti-infectious and can be of great help against influenza if they are used early enough: the sooner they are used after the onset of symptoms, the more likely they are to give a positive result. With the onset of a sore throat or fever, add the oils to water and use them as a gargle (*see* Aromatherapy Techniques). Try inhalations, a room vaporizer, aromatherapy baths, or direct application of the oils on to the body via a carrier lotion.

Preparing a multi-purpose treatment cream

It can be very useful to have a ready-mixed treatment to hand in case it is needed urgently. Choose an unperfumed base cream and add your choice of appropriate essential oils.

△ **1** Add a few drops of a self-prepared essential oil mix to your base cream. Use 5 drops of essential oil for every 50 ml base cream for a moisturizer.

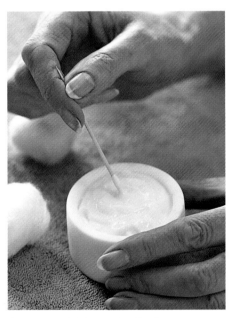

△ **2** Use a toothpick or the handle of a teaspoon to blend the oils into the cream. The prepared cream is ideal for use as a moisturizer or hand cream.

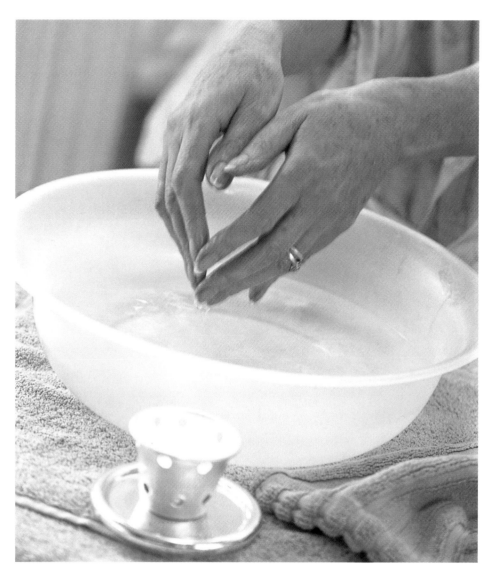

◁ If it is not possible to take a full aromatherapy bath, a hand or foot bath can be as effective for arthritic hands and feet. Add a few drops of your chosen oils to warm water and soak your hands for ten to fifteen minutes.

incontinence

This upsetting condition can be helped by gentle exercise to strengthen the pelvic floor muscles. Lying on your back, tense and relax your pelvic muscles, by raising your hips 10–20 times a day, at regular intervals. Astringent essential oils can also be useful, taken internally in a tea (*see* Aromatherapy Techniques).

pressure sores

If a woman becomes bed-bound she is at risk of developing pressure sores, which are notoriously difficult to heal. To prevent these, the patient should be moved every few hours so that she is not left too long in the same position. Rub a mix of essential oils in calendula into the buttock area every day. If weeping sores develop, prepare a mineral water mix (*see* Aromatherapy Techniques) with essential oils, shake well and use to spray on to the affected area.

digestive problems

There are two ways to treat upsetting digestive problems with aromatherapy. The most effective way to treat digestive disorders with essential oils is by ingestion (*see* Aromatherapy Techniques). Ideally, you should consult a qualified aromatologist. If you do decide to treat yourself, it is imperative to use only genuine essential oils from a reputable supplier and to carefully follow the directions in this book.

Application of recommended essential oils can also give good results. The oils can be mixed in a carrier lotion and rubbed gently on to the abdomen in a clockwise direction, or applied on a compress and left on the abdomen overnight.

indigestion

This can occur for a number of reasons: eating too much or too quickly, eating foods which are too rich, or through emotional causes such as worry, impatience and frustration. Essential oils are excellent for indigestion. Relevant essential oils can be used in an abdominal massage every 30 minutes before a meal.

constipation

This may arise as a side-effect of medication or through emotional causes, such as fear and anxiety. Changes in environment and routine can also bring on constipation.

diarrhoea

This may be due to anxiety, fear, infections, other medication or an overdose of laxatives taken to relieve constipation.

diverticulitis

Small, harmless, thin-walled sacs can form on the colon in elderly people, through insufficient fibre in the diet. Diverticulitis is when these sacs become inflamed and painful, leading to occasional bleeding and chronic constipation. Switch to a fibre-rich diet, and use essential oils for constipation and other anti-inflammatory conditions.

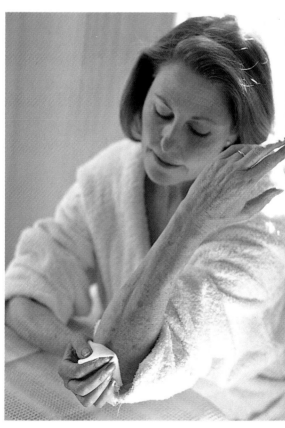

△ Lavender oil soaked into a warm compress can help to relieve the pain of arthritic joints.

Strengthening mental health

Physical health problems, minor or major, can become a source of worry and anxiety for an aging person, and can affect their overall mental and emotional health.

headaches and migraines

The reason for these, especially in the elderly, is not always apparent. It is therefore a good idea to use two or more essential oils, to make best use of their synergy. Put the relevant essential oils into your moisturizing cream and use twice daily. This helps both to relieve and prevent the problem, and will benefit the skin at the same time. If headaches persist throughout the day, try inhalation. If the headaches frequently recur, consider that it may be due to a food allergy, such as caffeine. If home treatment is unsuccessful it may be worth visiting a qualified aromatherapist.

shock

The emotional impact of shock can be particularly traumatic for an elderly person. Very often the shock is accompanied by fear, especially in the case of someone who lives on their own. Shock-induced trauma can be helped immediately by inhaling or applying essential oils with a sedative effect.

◁ **Oils for fear and anger can be a useful support for cancer patients. Use juniper, lemon and geranium in a base lotion and apply the mix to the hands and body.**

insomnia

Insomnia is fairly common amongst older people, and can get worse as age advances. Sometimes, there is no clear explanation for it – older people seem to need less sleep. However, the problem may be caused or exacerbated by anxiety and worry. Cramp in the leg muscles or arthritic pain during the night can also disturb the sleep pattern. The traditional essential oil used to help insomnia is lavender, although care should be taken with the dose, as too much will keep you wide awake. Lavender oil, used alone or in a synergy with two or three oils, has been used successfully by some hospitals to treat insomnia.

◁ **Lavender and sweet marjoram oils can help with grief and fear. Inhale them from a tissue.**

cancer

Aromatherapy cannot cure cancer but it can be used in a supportive role and can greatly improve the quality of life for many cancer patients. Fear of developing cancer can be a big worry for someone who has already lost a relative through the disease, and for cancer patients whose cancer is in remission. Use oils which are good for stress conditions (*see* Coping with Stress and Emotions), and apply by inhalation, compresses and direct application in a carrier lotion.

dementia

Some people, more often in old age, suffer deterioration of their mental faculties, and are unable to think clearly or to concentrate for any length of time. The memory can become unreliable and confused, and some

▷ Persistent headaches are debilitating and stressful. Massaging the shoulders with Roman chamomile and lavender will have a sedative and calming effect, while peppermint and rosemary will be energizing and uplifting.

speech difficulties may develop (this is particularly true after a stroke). Alzheimer's disease may develop if the nerve tissue (which cannot regenerate itself) withers and dies in the brain. Try using essential oils which stimulate the mind and improve memory. Some oils are also thought to be able to trigger past experiences, which is helpful for people with Alzheimer's.

Parkinson's disease

The cause of this debilitating, progressive disease is unknown, but a lack of the chemical substance, dopamine, which is needed for co-ordination of the brain muscles, seems to be responsible for its symptoms. Parkinson's disease is characterized by tremors, muscular rigidity and emaciation, and causes difficulty in speech and movement. Strong drugs are available to replace the dopamine; these help for a while, but they gradually lose efficiency as the body gets used to them. This necessitates a regular increase in dosage levels as the years pass, until, finally, the maximum dose loses its effect, and nothing more can be done to help the patient.

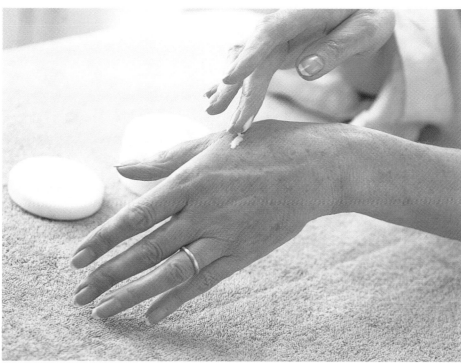

Side effects of the drugs include nausea, insomnia and constipation, all of which can be helped by aromatherapy. One study has also shown that essential oils can alleviate muscular problems, occasionally reducing the degree of slurred speech and tremors. Daily application of a lotion containing essential oils, plus daily aromatherapy baths (where possible) were used in the study. The symptoms which cause the most problems seem to be anxiety, lack of energy, muscular pains and stiffness. Others are constipation, insomnia, cramp, rigidity, tremors and slurred speech. Choose essential oils on the basis of the symptoms causing the trouble.

◁ For sufferers of Parkinson's disease, a hand and body lotion containing clary sage, sweet marjoram and rosemary can help the condition.

Useful essential oils

essential oil	treatment
poor circulation	
Clary sage *Salvia sclarea*	circulatory problems, haemorrhoids, varicose veins, venous aneurism, cholesterol
Lemon *Citrus limon*	poor circulation, thrombosis, varicose veins
Rosemary *Rosmarinus officinalis*	decongestant, poor circulation, hardening of the arteries
arthritis and rheumatism	
Chamomile (Roman) *Chamaemelum nobile*	anti-inflammatory, stress-relieving
Clove bud *Syzygium aromaticum*	analgesic (severe pain), anti-inflammatory, neurotonic (use sparingly - *see* The Essential Oils)
Lavender *Lavandula angustifolia*	analgesic, anti-inflammatory, stress-relieving
Marjoram (sweet) *Origanum majorana*	analgesic, stress-relieving
Niaouli *Melaleuca viridiflora*	analgesic, anti-inflammatory, neurotonic
Rosemary *Rosmarinus officinalis*	analgesic, anti-inflammatory, decongestant, neuromuscular action, neurotonic
bronchial asthma and bronchitis	
Marjoram (sweet) *Origanum majorana*	antispasmodic, anti-infectious, expels mucus, respiratory tonic
Niaouli *Melaleuca viridiflora*	anticatarrhal, anti-infectious, anti-inflammatory, expels mucus
Peppermint *Mentha* x *piperita*	anti-inflammatory, breaks down and expels mucus
Pine *Pinus sylvestris*	analgesic, anti-infectious, anti-inflammatory, decongestant, breaks down and expels mucus
Rosemary *Rosmarinus officinalis*	breaks down mucus, anti-inflammatory, decongestant, expels mucus
headaches	
Chamomile (Roman) *Chamaemelum nobile*	antispasmodic, calming, sedative
Lavender *Lavandula angustifolia*	analgesic, calming, sedative
Marjoram (sweet) *Origanum majorana*	analgesic, antispasmodic, calming
Melissa *Melissa officinalis*	calming, sedative
Peppermint *Mentha* x *piperita*	analgesic, antispasmodic
Rosemary *Rosmarinus officinalis*	analgesic, antispasmodic, decongestant

essential oil	treatment
influenza	
Eucalyptus *Eucalyptus smithii*	anti-infectious, antiviral, prophylactic
Cypress *Cupressus sempervirens*	anti-infectious
Lemon *Citrus limon*	anti-infectious, antiviral
Pine *Pinus sylvestris*	anti-infectious
insomnia	
Basil *Ocimum basilicum* var. *album*	nervous system regulator (nervous insomnia)
Chamomile (Roman) *Chamaemelum nobile*	calming
Lavender *Lavandula angustifolia*	calming, sedative
Lemon *Citrus limon*	calming
Marjoram (sweet) *Origanum majorana*	calming
Melissa *Melissa officinalis*	calming, sedative
shock	
Bergamot *Citrus bergamia*	balancing, calming, sedative, tonic to central nervous system
Chamomile (Roman) *Chamaemelum nobile*	calming, sedative
Lavender *Lavandula angustifolia*	balancing, calming, sedative, tonic
Melissa *Melissa officinalis*	calming, sedative
incontinence	
Cypress *Cupressus sempervirens*	astringent
Lemon *Citrus limon*	astringent
pressure sores	
Chamomile (German) *Matricaria recutica*	cicatrizant (infected wounds, ulcers)
Chamomile (Roman) *Chamaemelum nobile*	vulnerary (boils, burns wounds).
Frankincense *Boswellia carteri*	cicatrizant (scars, ulcers, wounds)
Geranium *Pelargonium graveolens*	cicatrizant (burns, cuts, ulcers, wounds)
Lavender *Lavandula angustifolia*	cicatrizant (burns, scars, varicose veins, wounds)
constipation and diverticulitis	
Ginger *Zingiber officinale*	analgesic, digestive stimulant, general tonic
Mandarin *Citrus reticulata*	antispasmodic, calming, digestive.
Orange (bitter) *Citrus aurantium* var. *amara*	calming, digestive

essential oil	treatment
Rosemary *Rosmarinus officinalis*	analgesic, anti-inflammatory, digestive (constipation, sluggish or painful digestion)

diarrhoea

essential oil	treatment
Geranium *Pelargonium graveolens*	anti-inflammatory (colitis), anti-spasmodic (colic, gastroenteritis), astringent
Lemon *Citrus limon*	antispasmodic, astringent, stomachic (gastritis, stomach ulcers).
Marjoram (sweet) *Origanum majorana*	analgesic, anti-infectious, anti-spasmodic (colic), stomachic (enteritis)
Niaouli *Melaleuca viridiflora*	anti-infectious, anti-inflammatory, antiviral (viral enteritis), digestive (gastritis)
Peppermint *Mentha x piperita*	anti-infectious, anti-inflammatory (colitis, enteritis, gastritis), antispasmodic (gastric spasm), digestive

indigestion (dyspepsia)

essential oil	treatment
Basil *Ocimum basilicum* var. *album*	analgesic, carminative (flatulence, sluggish digestion)
Lemon *Citrus limon*	digestive (nausea, painful digestion, flatulence, appetite loss)
Marjoram (sweet) *Origanum majorana*	analgesic, calming, digestive - (flatulence, indigestion)
Orange (bitter) *Citrus aurantium* var. *amara*	calming, digestive
Peppermint *Mentha x piperita*	analgesic, carminative (flatulence), digestive (nausea, painful digestion)
Rosemary *Rosmarinus officinalis*	analgesic (painful digestion), carminative (flatulence)

dementia and Alzheimer's disease

essential oil	treatment
Basil *Ocimum basilicum* var. *album*	neurotonic (mental strain)
Clove bud *Syzygium aromaticum*	mental stimulant (memory loss, mental fatigue), neurotonic
Marjoram (sweet) *Origanum majorana*	neurotonic (mental instability)
Peppermint *Mentha x piperita*	mental stimulant (concentration), neurotonic
Rosemary *Rosmarinus officinalis*	neurotonic (loss of memory, concentration)

Parkinson's disease

essential oil	treatment
Clary sage *Salvia sclarea*	antispasmodic, calming, regenerative (cellular aging), neurotonic
Lavender *Lavandula angustifolia*	analgesic, antispasmodic, calming, sedative (anxiety, headaches, insomnia), neurotonic
Marjoram (sweet) *Origanum majorana*	analgesic, antispasmodic, digestive tonic, calming (anxiety, insomnia),
Rosemary *Rosmarinus officinalis*	analgesic, antispasmodic, digestive (constipation, sluggish digestion), neurotonic

...'Tis the hour

That scatters spells on herb and flower

And garlands might be gathered now

That turn'd around the sleeper's brow.

From Light of the Haram, Thomas Moore, 1779–1852.

Ayurvedic Beauty

A tradition of beauty

Ayurveda, the "science of life", is a philosophy that covers every aspect of being: health, food, spirit, sex, occupation and relationships. It teaches how to live in harmony with your inner self and with the world around you. At one extreme of this far-reaching philosophy are the practices of religious ascetics, who subject themselves to fasts and other rigours to try to transcend the physical. At the other extreme are the sensual paintings, sculptures and writings that reveal a people at ease with their bodies and appreciative of the pleasures of life.

beauty of body and soul

For both men and women, beauty is seen as a blessing in India: gods and goddesses, heroes and heroines are depicted as handsome and graceful, with arched eyebrows and delicate features, and images of women's beauty and vigour appear in the earliest sacred texts. Traditionally, Indian women have adorned themselves with jewellery, make-up and body art. They have perfumed their hair and dressed it with flowers and gems. They have worn garments in dazzling colours, choosing fitted blouses that emphasize body shape, or swirling saris that draw attention to graceful movement.

Both sexes have traditionally groomed themselves to make the most of their looks. Since the earliest times, Ayurvedic remedies have included techniques to brighten eyes, clear skin and enhance the lustre of hair. Anti-aging treatments are among the most popular, aimed at restoring not only physical vigour but also a youthful appearance.

Because the philosophy of Ayurveda treats body, mind and soul as interrelated, beauty is not limited to the physical dimension, but reflects the vitality and health of the whole person, and adornment plays only a minor part. Jewels are valued not only for their beauty but also because they are considered to possess health-enhancing properties. Herbal remedies and treatments aim to cleanse the body from the

△ **Harmony is the essence of Ayurveda. India's goddesses of wisdom, love, life and death teach their followers to blend action with reflection, courage with compassion, so beauty grows from inner radiance.**

inside, while meditative practices prevent stress leaving its mark, and a fitness regime ensures agelessly youthful physical grace.

Ayurvedic medicine

Some of the basic principles of Ayurveda were set out more than 3,000 years ago in the Vedas, the sacred texts of Hinduism, and its teachings are believed to have been passed on by word of mouth for many centuries before that. The earliest medical textbooks, the *Susruta Samhita* and the *Charaka Samhita* (written before 500 BC and still consulted

today), list more than 700 herbal medicines, 125 surgical instruments and a range of procedures including cosmetic surgery and kidney-stone removal. Human bones excavated from the city of Harappa, dating from before 1500 BC, bear evidence of surgical repairs.

In the ancient world, Ayurveda's influence spread as far as Egypt, China and Greece. Since Western medicine developed from that of the ancient Greeks, a trace of Ayurveda survives in modern medical training, for example in kidney operations and the diagnosis of eye disease. In most ways, modern medicine has diverged from older traditions, focusing on symptoms and specific diseases, but now, when the healing power of antibiotics is waning because of overuse, and other wonder drugs have revealed harmful side-effects, the ancient wisdom of traditional holistic healing systems is again being sought. Western medicine is starting to open its mind, admitting that some treatments work in ways that no one understands and that mind and body can work together to heal illness.

Meanwhile, Ayurvedic researchers are publishing impressive results in mainstream medical journals. In one study, a remedy called gugalipid, made of resin from the myrrh tree, was found to lower cholesterol levels by an average of 20 per cent. In another, doctors reported that the skin condition of patients using an Ayurvedic remedy improved noticeably, while a placebo had no such results.

balance and harmony

The principle of Ayurveda is that good health stems from a correct balance of different energies and harmony with the outside world. As a medical system it is holistic, and though remedies exist for specific problems, they are varied according to the person.

▽ **A traditional exercise regime and an active lifestyle can allow every woman to achieve the natural grace of a classical dancer.**

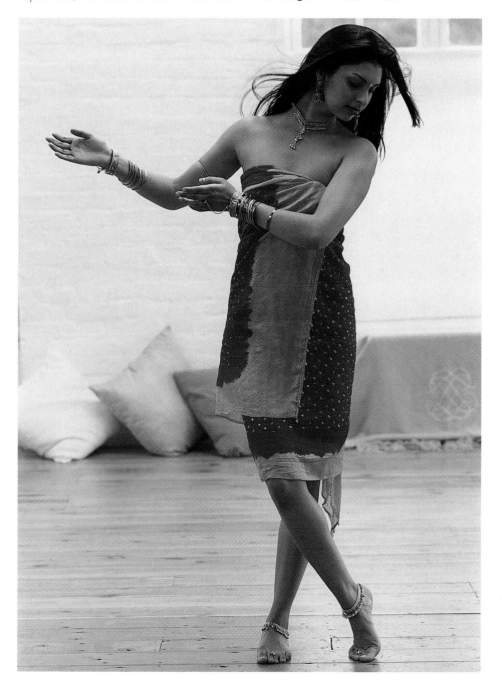

△ **Jewellery and ornament symbolize some of the links between the worlds of body and spirit.**

Ayurveda also works on levels other than the physical, and this is where it differs most radically from Western medicine. It is part of a world-view that accepts the existence of the unseen, both as part of a human being (a non-physical body that overlaps with the physical one) and as external energies that can affect us. Ayurveda makes no division between science and religion, so its medical system places at least as much emphasis on the psychological and spiritual as on the physical. Most treatments are intended to bring disturbed energies back into balance, allowing the body to heal itself.

△ **Prayer and meditation may help as much as herbal remedies when health disorders indicate that vital energies have been disturbed.**

Living energies, healing powers

△ **Fire is one of the five elemental forces present in the whole of creation, including ourselves.**

According to Ayurveda, five *mahabhutas* or "great elements" – air, fire, water, earth, and ether (or space) – constitute the world with everything in it, including ourselves, and they affect us through three primary forces called *doshas* (meaning "flaws"): *vata*, *pitta* and *kapha*. Each dosha owes its character to the elements associated with it:

• Vata, linked with the elements air and ether, is dry. It governs movement of every kind, both mental and physical.

• Pitta, linked with fire and water, is hot. It governs all the processes of change and transformation, such as digestion.

• Kapha, linked with earth and water, is heavy. It governs structure and stability.

channels of energy

The doshas are not the only forces that affect us, because our non-physical body has its own detailed anatomy. Just as the blood carries oxygen around the body, another equally essential life force called *prana* circulates in channels of its own. At any junction – for example where two kinds of tissue meet, such as bone and tendon, or where the influences of two energies meet – there are *marma points*, where energy sometimes gets blocked. One of the major

energy channels follows the line of the backbone and is studded with seven important points called *chakras*.

The physical and non-physical constantly overlap. For example, *ama*, a toxin formed in the body, can be created by poorly digested food or by an experience you can't assimilate – or swallow. *Ojas*, the subtle energy that connects body, mind and spirit, both creates our aura and underpins the immune system. It is formed from the seven kinds of body tissue, and is also influenced by meditation.

imbalance

We are born in a state called *prakruti*, with all three doshas in balance though not in equal amounts. Each of us is governed by one more than the others, and our individual natures mean that even with the energies comfortably in balance, we'll show the attributes of the dominant dosha. Problems begin when one dosha becomes excessively powerful, pushing us to extremes of behaviour or creating ill-health. Excessive vata might cause anxiety or a hacking cough. Too much fiery pitta could trigger an attack of road rage or heartburn.

Stolid kapha could bring everything to a standstill, resulting in anything from lethargy to blocked sinuses. To prevent or remedy such problems, Ayurveda aims to maintain balance in all things. That includes keeping people in harmony with their surroundings and with each other, keeping bodily processes working effectively, and keeping body, mind and spirit integrated.

Sometimes imbalance results from an excess of one of the doshas, perhaps because we're eating the wrong kinds of food. Or we could be affected by something we've come into contact with, since everything has one of three *gunas*, or inner qualities: harmonious *sattva*, aggressive *rajas* or dull *tamas*. Anything from foods to colours to thoughts will do us good if it's sattvic, but is likely to cause irritation if it's rajasic or heaviness if it's tamasic. The problem could even be caused by karma: the result of misdeeds in this life or a previous one.

Ayurvedic therapies

All Ayurvedic treatment is aimed at restoring balance, in order to keep us strong enough – both in spirit and in immune system – to withstand disease, so it is used for

△ **To locate the crown marma point, rest one hand on the bridge of your nose and measure three fingerwidths back from your fingertips.**

△ **Massage this point to get blocked energy moving on if you are suffering from a feeling of confusion.**

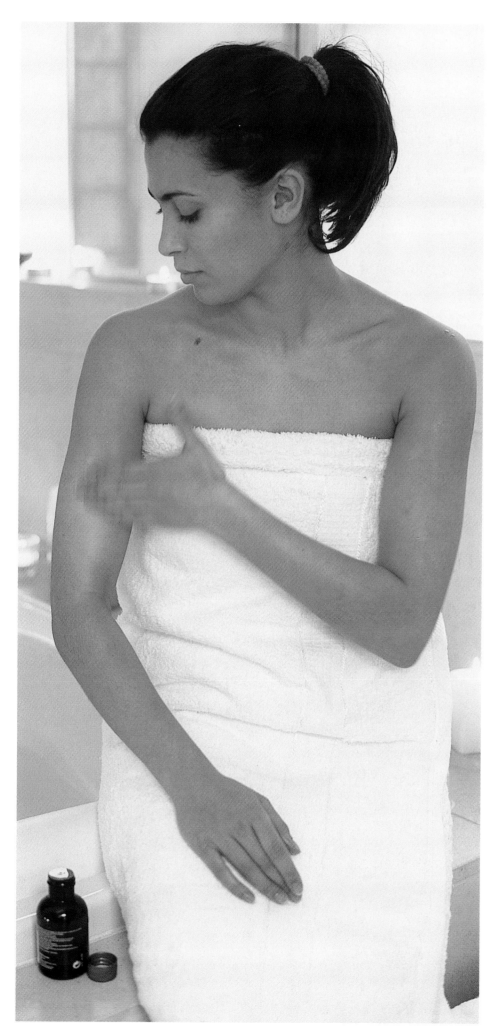

▷ Ayurveda recommends regular detoxifying treatments, starting with steam baths and herbal oil massage. Spring is a good time to initiate these cleansing practices.

prevention as well as for cure. Massage, yoga and meditation form part of Ayurveda's recommended daily routine, but can also be used to treat certain health problems.

Nutrition is one of Ayurveda's central elements, with the emphasis not only on wholesome ingredients but also on the right foods for you as an individual. Each dosha can be aggravated by certain foods, so if you're suffering from an imbalance, you'll be urged to avoid those foods and eat others that have a calming effect.

Detoxification, or *shodhana*, begins with *purvakarma*: cleansing steam baths and herbal oil massages. Then comes *panchakarma*, a more rigorous detox that may include enemas, laxatives, and nasal washes with herbs or oils. In case blocked energy is causing congestion, the marma points may be stimulated to encourage the flow. This is usually done with finger pressure, though needles may also be used.

The next step, *rasayana*, aims to restore long-term health and slow down the aging process through lifestyle changes, meditation and exercises, with herbal remedies if necessary. A course of treatment may last for up to six months.

Though some of Ayurveda's practices seem strenuous, it's a compassionate philosophy that understands human desires and aims to increase the quality of life, promoting vitality and inner harmony.

△ Hand massage stimulates the marma points that are clustered in this area, and it is easy to do it for yourself.

Dosha analysis

If you consult an Ayurvedic doctor you may be asked to complete a questionnaire to find out your *prakruti* – your constitution, determined at the time of your birth – and your current imbalance, or *vikruti*. The questionnaire is part of a package of diagnostic tools; others include checking your pulses (subtle energy flows) and examining the condition of your tongue. Answering a questionnaire at home can give you an idea of your vikruti, as your answers will usually be based on your current condition, but it does not replace a full consultation with a practitioner.

You may find that more than one description applies to you. In this case, tick all that are relevant. In the skin and hair sections, respond only to the descriptions that apply to you. Give yourself plenty of time to think before answering, so your answers will be as accurate as possible.

◁ Completing a questionnaire can give some insight into your current needs, so make sure your answers reflect the way you're feeling right now.

▷ To discover your true constitution – the state in which you were born – you'll need to consult an Ayurvedic practitioner. The results may surprise you.

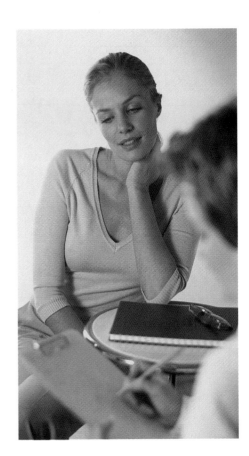

dosha analysis

PHYSICAL TRAITS	VATA	PITTA	KAPHA
Body frame	Thin	Medium	Large
Fingernails	Thin/cracking	Pink/soft/medium	Thick/wide/pale
Weight	Low/bony	Medium/muscular	Gains easily
Stool/bowel movement	Small/hard/wind	Loose/burning	Moderate/solid
Forehead size	Small	Medium	Large
Appetite	Variable	Strong	Constant
Eyes	Small/unsteady	Reddish/focused	Wide/white
Voice	Low or weak	High or sharp	Slow or quiet
Lips	Cracking, thin, dry	Medium or soft	Large or smooth
Speech	Quick or talkative	Moderate or argumentative	Deep or melodious
Weather: what bothers you?	Cold and dry	Heat and sun	Cold and damp
Sleep patterns	Light	Moderate	Deep/heavy
Which do you like best?	Travel or nature	Sports or politics	Water or flowers

MENTAL TRAITS	VATA	PITTA	KAPHA
Temperament	Nervous or fearful	Irritable or impatient	Easy-going
Memory	Quickly grasps, but forgets	Sharp or clear	Slow to learn, never forgets
Faith	Radical or changing	Leader- or goal-oriented	Loyal or constant
Dreams	Flying or anxious	Fighting or in colour	Few or romantic
Emotions	Enthusiastic or worried	Warm or angry	Calm or attached
Mind	Quick or adaptable	Penetrating or critical	Slow and steady

SKIN TENDENCIES	VATA	PITTA	KAPHA
	Lack of tone or lustre	Rashes, inflammation, itching	Dull, sluggish, congested
	Rough patches	Oily T-zone	Enlarged pores
	Chapping and cracking	Premature wrinkling	Large pustules
	Dry eczema	Blackheads	Cystic formations
	General dryness	General excessive oiliness	Thick, oily secretions
	Dandruff/dry scalp	Discoloration	Oily scalp
	Fine, porcelain	Warm, smooth	Strong, flawless

HAIR	VATA	PITTA	KAPHA
	Dry and dull	Oily	Thick
	Frizzy	Balding	Glossy
	Scaly scalp	Excessive hair loss	Shiny
	Split ends	Thinning	Grows easily

▽ Vata is a fine, light, speedy energy that can cause problems with dryness of skin and hair.

▽ If pitta's fiery warmth slips out of balance, it may express itself in rashes and discoloration.

▽ Kapha's strong skin and thick hair age slowly; excess oiliness is the main beauty pitfall.

Your dosha and you

Few people are ruled by a single dosha. Most of us are governed by dual doshas, one of which is more powerful than the other. A very few are ruled equally by all three.

If your score in the questionnaire is highest in pitta but still quite high in kapha, for example, that makes you a pitta-kapha combination. Scores reversed for pitta and kapha would make you a kapha-pitta. The pitta-kapha person is more likely to suffer from a pitta imbalance than anything else. But a combination of factors that aggravate kapha – such as eating a lot of heavy food during a cold, damp spring – could produce an excess of kapha energy.

self-analysis

The results of the questionnaire can be enlightening. If they are puzzling because they seem unlike you, your answers to the questions may not have been completely accurate: perhaps you overstated your faults or gave answers you felt ought to be true. You may be used to thinking of yourself in a way that is no longer relevant.

△ **Morning is the best time for meditation, when peaceful kapha energy helps to still your mind.**

◁ **Vata dominates the afternoon hours, making this a good time for thought and intellectual activity, rather than physical work.**

Comparisons should be made with other people of your own ethnic background, not against some kind of world average. Kapha, for example, tends to go with fair skin and vata with dark skin. But a typical kapha person from Sri Lanka would be darker than, say, a typical vata from Sweden.

Remember too that your mind and body may be ruled by different doshas, so you might have a fiery pitta temperament in a curvy kapha body. All kinds of external factors can affect you: even the season or weather could influence your answers. So don't feel ruled by the results you obtain. They are meant to offer guidance, not lay down the law.

In order to discover your prakruti, or constitutional dosha, an Ayurvedic practitioner will carry out a pulse analysis, taking the pulses of the subtle energy flows at 21 points. The difference between your prakruti and your vikruti can be revealing. Prakruti is your ideal state, with everything in the best balance for your personality – if there's a big difference it could mean you're living in a way that doesn't suit you.

what is an imbalance?

We all have one or two doshas that dominate. It's natural for each of us to show some characteristics of these, whether they are most noticeable in our looks, behaviour or tastes. The doshas also give us warning of what needs to be tackled if something goes wrong with our well-being.

When a dominant dosha becomes excessively strong, its characteristics are exaggerated. As a pitta type you will be naturally ambitious and competitive, for example, but if pitta grows too strong you may become irritable and critical, and have trouble sleeping. This is known as a pitta imbalance. If you don't tackle an imbalance

THE DOSHAS THROUGH THE DAY	
6am–10am	Kapha
10am–2pm	Pitta
2pm–6pm	Vata
6pm–10pm	Kapha
10pm–2am	Pitta
2am–6am	Vata

early on, it can eventually manifest itself in sickness, so you need to reduce your dominant dosha. In this case, that means cutting down on things like spicy food and dance music, which fuel pitta.

a time for everything

According to Ayurvedic teaching, each period of the day is ruled by a different energy, which can reinforce or counteract the influence of your dominant dosha.

Tranquil kapha governs early morning, the time for meditation. Later in the morning is the time to exercise, combining kapha strength with pitta energy. Pitta, which aids digestion, rules midday, making that the best time to eat. Vata dominates the afternoon – an ideal time for mental work, as vata promotes intelligence. Then come the quiet kapha hours again, making this the best time to get to sleep. Pitta takes over again after 10pm, when its fiery energy is meant to stop your temperature dropping too low while you sleep. If you go to bed after 10pm, you may find that a new rush of pitta-fuelled energy stops you dropping off.

▽ **Ayurveda advocates "early to bed, early to rise". Before 10pm, kapha helps you to get to sleep – after that, pitta could keep you awake.**

◁ **Pitta energy, which aids digestion, is in full force around lunchtime, making this the best time to enjoy your main meal of the day.**

The seasons follow the same rhythm as the hours of the day, with kapha ruling the weeks from spring to early summer, pitta ruling high summer and autumn, and vata rising when the leaves have fallen to dominate the winter.

Since an excess of any dosha brings out its harmful side, watch out for signs of an imbalance, especially during the times or seasons that correspond with your own dominant dosha. You might find it hard to drag yourself out of bed in the kapha-ruled morning, or that pitta's summer heat brings you out in a rash, or that you're getting stressed under vata's influence during the winter months. Medical researchers have found that seasonal affective disorder, or "winter blues", actually affects most people during spring, when depressive kapha is coming into force.

Even our own lives follow these phases. As children we are ruled by kapha, as adults pitta takes over and with the onset of wise old age we come into our vata time.

ESSENTIAL FLAWS

Why are the forces of vata, pitta and kapha called doshas, or "flaws"? Ayurveda takes the very practical view that, though everything ought to exist in perfect balance, it usually doesn't. Our individual natures dictate that one dosha will generally be dominant, and this is fine when it is just enough to express your individual personality, but when it becomes too strong and overrules the others, it throws your constitution out of balance, which leads to ill health. So a healthy life is one in which we manage to keep the balance steady.

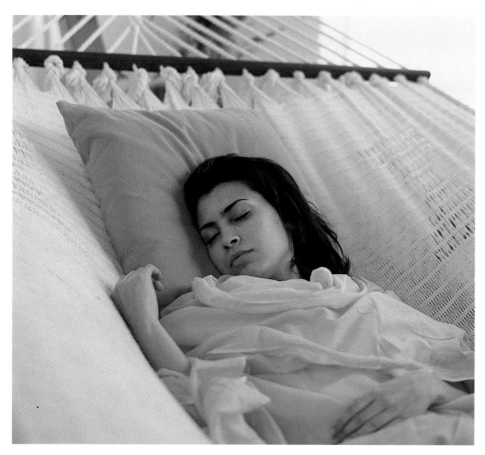

Vata movement and life force

Slender, willowy and long-legged, the classic vata woman looks good on a catwalk. She's more likely to be either tall or petite than of medium height. Her cool, porcelain skin is rarely bothered by spots or oily patches. Her rather small eyes sparkle with life and intelligence, and her fine hair complements her delicate bone structure.

She never thinks about her weight – she's naturally light. Her active lifestyle keeps her in shape, and she doesn't tend to eat a lot. She'd rather be in a club, dancing until dawn, than wasting time in a restaurant where you can't move to the music. Though a born athlete, she rarely builds a lot of muscle, but remains slim and slightly ethereal-looking.

as free as the air

Vata women love change, travel and movement. They're fast – whether they're running for the sheer joy of it or tackling some new concept in a physics class. They talk rapidly and their quick intellects mean they're full of ideas, plans and theories.

At work, vatas are the ones with all the ideas who'll get any project under way with the force of their enthusiasm, though they may not be so good at seeing it through: while someone with a steadier dosha takes over, they'll be hatching a dozen new plans. They're highly creative and often artistic, so no one really expects them to be utterly practical. They'd be exhausting company if they weren't so stimulating, but they rarely stay long enough to wear out their welcome.

vata imbalance

No one can keep up that pace for ever. Vatas are smart enough to know this, but often don't slow down until they've built up a massive vata imbalance by doing all the things that aggravate this ethereal dosha. These include skipping meals, not getting enough sleep and generally running themselves into the ground.

When vatas finally crash they may have trouble getting up again. Then they suffer

△ **Soothing oils do more than just nourish dry skin: they can help pacify excess vata energy.**

from stress and exhaustion, probably compounded by insomnia. Living on their nerves, they can forget to eat or may feel too anxious to swallow anything. Their rapid intellect can spin off into confusion. Tension can lead to muscle pain, cramps and irritable bowel syndrome. Excessive weight loss can also lead to serious health problems such as osteoporosis.

Dryness is the essential vata attribute, so an excess of vata causes dehydration in everything: hair and fingernails become brittle, lips crack, the tongue feels like felt, the eyes are sore. Dry skin conditions such as

◁ Listening to classical music with a slow, rhythmic beat can help to calm a vata imbalance, easing away feelings of tension and anxiety.

eczema can be a problem. A dry cough adds to the feeling of debility. Internal dryness can cause arthritis and constipation and even thicken the blood – add this to vata's raised stress levels, and it's not surprising that high blood pressure and heart palpitations are vata complaints.

pacifying vata

This dosha needs help to become more grounded. Pacifying influences are warm, moist, slow and contained. If you're vata, you're drawn towards speed, lightness, novelty. Try to balance these with activities that slow and centre you. Take a relaxing spa break instead of a strenuous activity holiday and discover the steam room and the jacuzzi. Listen to peaceful New Age or classical music. Find a course in meditation, then practise it at home some mornings instead of heading for the gym for your normal workout.

You like being with people, but this doesn't have to be in a crowded club. Invite friends around for supper instead. Take your time selecting wonderful ingredients, cooking the meal to perfection and eating it with people who care about you. Relax and enjoy the warmth of their company.

Cold, dry, windy weather makes you tense, so cocoon yourself away from it when

you can, and take your holidays on a tropical beach. Even the scents you use can fuel or calm your dosha: jasmine, sandalwood and rose all help to keep vata in balance.

your beauty needs

Dry skin is the classic vata complaint. The fine texture of your skin looks good when vata is in balance, but an imbalance makes it dull and lifeless. This kind of skin ages easily, so moisturizing is vital: the Ayurvedic way is to drink lots of water and eat plenty of the juicy fruits that help to pacify vata. Putting on weight isn't a problem for this dosha, so

you should never really need to count any calories, but you do need to beware of letting your weight fall too low.

Vata's flyaway hair is prone to dandruff, so a weekly sesame oil massage will relieve your dry scalp as well as easing tension. Teeth are a weak spot, exacerbated by the vata tendency to graze instead of eating meals, leaving teeth constantly coated in acid. If you can't cut out the snacks, rinse your mouth with water after every one.

▽ As a vata, you love company, and a leisurely meal with a friend will help you relax.

Pitta fire and transformation

Pitta woman is a dazzler. Fire is her dominant element, and it shows. Women of this dosha radiate energy like the sun, and their skin reflects their emotions with a surge of colour. Yet pitta also includes an element of water, which can stop this dosha burning out.

Despite a healthy appetite, pittas rarely become overweight. You're likely to spot them at the gym, where their powerful workouts result in toned muscles that curve rather than bulking up. They are usually blessed with soft hair, neat noses and small chins, and may have numerous beauty spots in the form of moles and freckles.

Though they're likely to have combination skin – with an oilier T-zone of forehead, nose and mouth – as long as pitta remains in balance the skin should be neither too dry nor too oily, but smooth and warm to the touch. Pittas often have warm, coppery skin tones.

fiery energies

The heat extends to the pitta character. Passionate and ambitious, pitta women know what they want and will strive to achieve it. They may fly off the handle, but

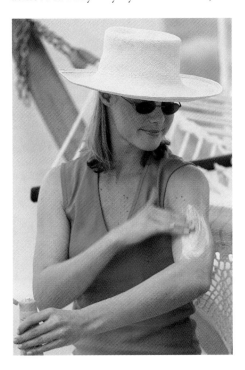

they're not the sort to hide a simmering grievance behind a mask of friendliness. Don't be fooled by this fiery image, though. As long as pitta remains in balance, they are intelligent, calm and rational. Born leaders, their qualities reward those who are drawn to their fire.

At work, they're high-fliers, strong-minded and focused: if they're enthusiastic about a project they'll see it through. They aim for the heights of success and often reach them, thanks to the single-minded work they put into getting there.

pitta imbalance

When pitta energy boils over, the heat is on. Rashes, inflammation, sweating, fevers and heartburn are all signs of a pitta imbalance, as are acne eruptions and hot flushes, which characterize the beginning and end of the fertile life period ruled by this fiery dosha.

A pitta imbalance will often reveal itself through the skin, in blotching or changes in pigmentation, or the flushing caused by indigestion. More serious ailments may be signalled by a yellowish complexion: this could be caused by liver dysfunction, which needs medical attention.

Fiery mood swings may be caused by another of pitta's problems – hormone imbalances. An excess of pitta can make someone overambitious, temperamental, jealous, aggressive and likely to trample on anyone in their path.

pacifying pitta

Your inner fire provides all the heat you need. Sultry weather and overheated buildings can provoke a pitta imbalance. When you go to the gym, head for the swimming pool rather than the sauna or hot tub. On holiday, go for the snow. In the summer, slow down to keep cool. The

◁ **Use sunscreen at all times to protect yourself from the sun (and be sure to avoid sunbeds), especially if you have moles or freckles.**

△ **If excessive pitta energy makes you irritable, soothe yourself with gentle influences: the scent of a gardenia, the sound of trickling water.**

influences that pacify excess pitta are cool, soft, kind and generally calming. The smell of gardenias is meant to cool pitta energy.

Give yourself time to eat breakfast and lunch sitting down, instead of skipping meals and overdosing on food in the evening. This can help you to avoid the pitta pitfalls of insomnia and indigestion, which add to your stress.

Avoid harsh or aggressive music, or anything with a driving beat or lots of drumming. Try soothing music with a slowish beat and gentle, minor chords.

Since high-tech equipment also increases pitta energy, an overheated office can cause problems. Freelance work can be one solution, keeping you away from office politics. On the other hand, being part of a team could help control your tendency to overwork. Whichever you choose, keep an eye on your stress levels and remember there's a world outside work. Cultivate friends who help you relax rather than contacts who can advance your career. Use some of your abundant creativity to express your artistic gifts, and divert some energy into working for a good cause that gives you a feelgood buzz.

your beauty needs

Ruled by fire, your skin reacts readily to inner or outer heat. You flush when you are angry and blush with embarrassment. Indigestion may give you an unwanted glow, and hot conditions make you look and feel uncomfortable. Colour-reducing foundation creams were made for you.

Your skin is sensitive, and a pitta imbalance can bring you out in rashes, rosacea, acne or – in later life – blotchy liver spots. Dark-skinned pittas sometimes suffer from pigmented patches. Your most important beauty rule is to keep cool. A mineral-water spray lives in your handbag or desk drawer; at home, cucumber makes an instant skin-cooling mask. Treat your skin kindly, avoiding harsh treatments that could bring it out in a rash.

Your skin isn't dry and shouldn't age too fast, as long as you protect it from the sun. It's lucky that pitta's sensitive skin and dislike of heat tend to stop you sunbathing, because you're more prone than anyone else to skin cancer. Keep an eye on all those moles, reporting any changes to your doctor.

A pitta imbalance can also affect your hair, making it prematurely thin and grey. Ayurvedic hair care aims at keeping the scalp healthy and strengthening growth.

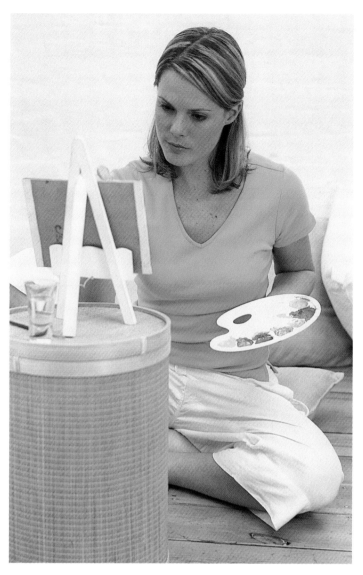

◁ To keep your life in balance, put some of your abundant pitta energy into expressing your natural creativity.

▽ Calm pitta heat with a refreshing spray of cool water – it's good for your skin, and for your equilibrium – or, even better, go for a swim.

Kapha growth and protection

A classic kapha type has perfect teeth, full lips and a flawless complexion, surrounded by masses of shining hair. But her greatest beauty shines out through her eyes, which are large, deep and thickly fringed with long eyelashes. The inner quality they reveal is one of peace and serenity. Kapha's very presence is calming, and the stress that aggravates vata's dizziness and pitta's temper seems to dissipate when a kapha person takes over. This is a peaceful, stable energy, combining earth's strength with water's deep stillness. Kapha people relax easily and rarely experience a troubled night.

▷ **Sensual kaphas appreciate the pleasures of food, but this can lead to weight gain. Spicy soups and curries will satisfy your tastebuds and pacify excess kapha energy.**

peace from earth

Calm and tolerant, kaphas are natural peace-makers. They make friends easily, love deeply and are wise enough to forgive things that would offend others. They happily nurture those they love, and frequently all those around them too, maintaining deep, rewarding relationships of all kinds. They are outstanding homemakers, and will go to great lengths to avoid change or upheaval.

At work they defuse tense situations with their down-to-earth good humour. In fact, tension is less likely to develop when there are kapha people around to carry a burden, because they are both physically and psychologically strong, with legendary powers of endurance. On a practical level, they'll finish the work that airy vatas started and lost interest in – and they won't be drawn into arguments with a bossy pitta. Good memory, aided by their natural patience, helps them stay on course and get the details right.

All sorts of people are drawn towards kapha's sweetness and warmth. Kaphas are too kind to reject anyone, but they have to beware of a tendency to let more demanding types take advantage.

kapha imbalance

In excess, grounded kapha energy can become heavy and stagnant. Kapha people relax very easily, and have to battle with their lazy tendencies. When kapha starts to overrule everything else, it's hard to get them off the sofa.

Exercise is vital to keep kapha energy at a healthy level, but lethargy may be a sign of another characteristic problem: depression. A kapha person in low spirits will tend to stay at home eating chocolate in front of the television: negative traits combining to increase the imbalance.

Groundedness can also distort into materialism, and when that happens, greed

◁ **Lethargy can be a problem for kaphas, especially when they are bored or lonely.**

Kaphas have to push themselves to exercise, but the ease with which they develop muscles is encouraging. They also need to work on flexibility and lightness.

and envy are kapha's less appealing traits, along with a possessive attachment to material things. A kapha overdose has a blunting, dulling effect on mental faculties, leading to obstinacy and narrow-mindedness. Physically, it is associated with sluggish digestion, constipation, respiratory congestion, diabetes, coronary artery disease, slowed metabolism and obesity.

pacifying kapha

You probably love rich food, sweet or savoury, and plenty of it. But that increases kapha energy as well as your hip measurement. If you're becoming greedy or sluggish, try some hot, spicy food for a change, and eat a bit less. Brisk scents such as cedar or camphor can sometimes help, as does anything that has a tendency to lighten, warm or invigorate.

Kapha people need to get up early and take daily exercise. If you're sleeping more than eight hours a night (nine in your teens), get your doctor to check for an underactive thyroid gland. Depression can also make you oversleep; to break the cycle, find an activity you can enjoy in company: team sports, walking or aerobics classes with a friend.

You need to stay stimulated, so seek new experiences and motivate yourself to go out to evening classes or art galleries. Put aside your cookbook and read a history of your

area, a thriller (make sure you solve the mystery before it's all revealed), or a biography of someone you admire.

Coldness increases kapha, so work up a sweat in the gym and enjoy the sauna too – not the steam room, because you need dry heat. Slap on the sunscreen and go out on sunny days. Take an outdoor holiday visiting archaeological sites in the North African

desert or exploring the Australian outback. Let your nurturing tendencies do yourself some good and adopt an unwanted dog: you're too kind-hearted to neglect the long walks it'll need.

your beauty needs

Kaphas have the sort of strong, smooth skin that shrugs off most blemishes and goes on to age well. Your idea of a bad-hair day would win no sympathy from anyone else.

What you have to watch out for is your weight. You're naturally strong and fit, so the health benefits of exercise aren't much of a draw. You enjoy life's little indulgences, such as good food, warmth and relaxation. A run down to the gym on a cold night sounds as much fun to you as drilling your own teeth.

The strongest of the doshas, you build muscle easily, so you'll see easy gains when you start working out. You'll need to cut down your fuel intake as well. But if you eat at the right time – just long enough before exercise to give you the energy you need without risking indigestion – you'll find working out doesn't make you overeat in compensation. Then your honed physique will start to offer its own rewards.

◁ Generous kaphas are the world's best cooks and decorators, with large circles of friends. They make wonderful party hosts.

Cleansing the Body, Clearing the Mind

Ayurveda aims to promote natural beauty and lifelong
youthfulness by keeping all the systems in balance.
The first essential is to clear the systems of
anything that hinders this aim. In physical
terms, it includes cleansing treatments
such as massage, steam therapy and
fasting. For the mind and spirit it
means discarding old habits of
thought that clutter up
the consciousness.

Healing hands

Massage plays a central role in Ayurvedic treatments, stimulating circulation and promoting the elimination of waste. Different versions are used to treat illness, heal injuries, aid detoxification, calm the mind, beautify the skin and rejuvenate the body. These treatments can now be found at Ayurvedic centres worldwide.

Abhyanga is the classic full-body massage, carried out by one or two therapists. As well as stroking and kneading movements, the therapists apply finger or hand pressure to some of the body's 107 marma points.

Champissage is a specialized head massage that stimulates marma points across the head, aiming to tone up all the body's systems. It helps to improve circulation, boost the immune system and slow down the aging process.

Shirodhara consists of pouring warm oil slowly on to your forehead while a therapist massages it gently into your scalp.

Pottali or **Navrakhizi** is a massage with hot poultices of rice, oil, milk and herbs. The resulting paste is washed off and more oil is massaged in. Traditionally used to treat vata conditions, it's as beneficial for stress and anxiety as for bodily aches.

Sarvangadhara or **Pizhichil** requires three therapists. One keeps a constant supply of oil warmed while two others dip linen cloths into the oil and squeeze it over the entire body, massaging it in lightly. This is a rejuvenating treatment that also aims to build up the immune system.

oil essentials

In Ayurvedic practice, oil is believed to help clear toxic ama out of the body. It also reduces excess dosha, which is considered to stick like a solid substance until softened and flushed out in the form of bodily secretions. Oil should be washed off after a treatment, so any waste products released into it don't re-enter the body.

MASSAGE FOR YOUR DOSHA

All dosha types benefit from massage. Vata people, and others who have dry skin, should always use oil for massage. The pitta dosha can be over-stimulated if too much oil is used, so just enough should be applied to avoid dragging the skin. Any kind of massage helps to provide the stimulation a kapha body requires, but deep-tissue massage is especially useful in aiding waste disposal via the lymph system.

You can choose an oil purely because it is suitable for your skin type. But if you feel that you are suffering from an excess of one of your energies – light-headed vata, for example, or impatient pitta – choose an appropriate oil for your dosha. Take outside influences into account: if it's a damp evening in spring, for example, kapha energy will already be high.

Full body self-massage

Ayurveda recommends self-massage each morning. As you do it, vary your touch so that you're sometimes moving your hands lightly over the skin, and at other times pressing firmly enough to move the skin over the bone. Use the fingertips for static pressure, but the softer pads of the fingers for kneading or circling movements. Avoid putting pressure on any joints. Unless otherwise stated, any pressure should be upward, towards the head. Always warm the oil, and make sure the room is pleasantly warm. Start by pouring a little oil into one palm and rubbing your hands together. Repeat from time to time as the oil wears off your hands. If you prefer not to get oil in your hair, you can do the head massage without it.

△ **1** Press your hands against your scalp and move the skin in large circles. Run your fingers through your hair and gently tug and rotate small sections of it to stimulate the scalp. With the tips of your fingers and thumbs, make little circles all over your head.

△ **2** Smooth oil into your neck and work it up over the back of your head. Cup the base of the skull in your palms and press gently upwards.

△ **3** Run well-oiled palms in long strokes up your throat from the collarbones, covering the front and the sides; repeat several times.

△ **4** Cupping your chin in each palm alternately, run the fingers up along the jawline to the ears several times, using firm pressure without dragging the skin.

△ **5** Place your thumbs on your temples and massage the forehead in small circles with your fingertips. Use light pressure, and keep the movement upward and outward. Massage the cheeks in the same way.

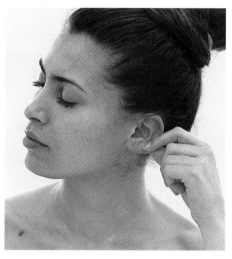

△ **6** Continue massaging in small circles all over the scalp and along the base of the skull. Gently pull and twist sections of the hair to stimulate the scalp. Then rub and squeeze the ears and massage all around them.

△ **7** Relax your head and shoulders and let your head sink forwards, keeping your shoulders down. Place your oiled palms on the back of your neck and rub firmly from the spine out to the sides.

△ **8** Rub oil into each shoulder with large circular motions, using your whole palm and fingers. If you have any stiffness, cup your hand around the joint and rotate it as far as you find comfortable.

△ **9** Stroke oil outwards across your chest from your breastbone. Pull the fingers outwards in a semicircular movement, from the nipples towards the armpits, both above and below the breasts.

△ **10** Extend one arm, thumb upwards, and stroke lightly down the outside of the arm with your palm. Then reverse the movement and rub more firmly back up the inside of the arm.

continued over page ▷

11 Grip your left arm just below the shoulder (▷), squeezing it between your fingers and the heel of your right hand. Move your hand a couple of fingers' width down your arm and repeat, working your way down to the hand. With the left hand extended, palm down, massage the wrist and the back of the hand (△) with the right hand. Grip and release the side of the wrist (▽). Repeat, working down the side of the hand to the fingertips.

△ **12** Hold the left hand and massage the palm with your right thumb (above left). Now squeeze and massage each finger, finishing by pulling it gently (above right). Interlace your fingers and stretch the arms out in front of you, palms facing outwards. Keep your shoulders relaxed and low. Release your grip. Turning your left palm down, rub briskly up from the back of your hand to the shoulder. Repeat the arm and hand massage on the right.

CURING OIL

Oil for Ayurvedic massage is traditionally "cured" before use. To cure oil, pour it into an enamelled or non-metallic pan, add a drop of water and place over a gentle heat until the water pops, then remove from the stove. When cool, pour the oil into a glass bottle and store away from light. Just before a massage, warm a little of the oil to a comfortable temperature.

◁ **13** Reach over each shoulder with your fingers pointing downwards. Rub as far as you can stretch down and across your back, and press your fingers in as you pull back up, feeling that you are stretching the muscles upwards.

△ **14** With fingers pointing downwards, massage your abdomen with the flat of your hands in large clockwise movements, above and below the navel. If you suffer from poor digestion, you may massage with your fist, slowly circling down on the left and up on the right. Finish by stroking outwards from the centre.

△ **15** Reaching behind your waist, put your hands flat on your lower back, with fingertips on the spine, and draw them out to the sides, pressing firmly. Massage your hips and buttocks briskly with kneading, pummelling and large circular stroking movements, being careful to avoid direct pressure on your hip joints.

△ **16** Lightly rub oil down your legs, then massage up the calf muscles. Grip and release, or rub firmly in circles with fists spiralling upwards, or simply stroke firmly up towards the knees. If you have varicose or visible veins, stroke gently without any pressure.

△ **17** Work gently over each knee, rubbing the kneecap, sides and back of the leg in circles using plenty of oil. Then stroke vigorously up the insides of the thighs, with brisk overlapping movements, into the groin.

18 Massage your feet one at a time. To begin, cup the heel in one hand and, with the other hand, grasp the toes and gently rotate the foot (△ above left) in both directions. Massage lightly over the ankle and top of the foot in circles, using more pressure on the sole to avoid tickling. Gently rotate each toe (△ above right). Finish by stroking firmly down from the ankle several times as if brushing something off the ends of the toes (▽).

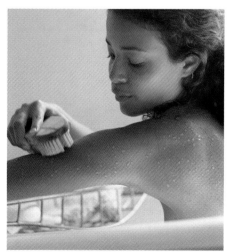

A TOUCH OF SILK

The full-body massage can be done without oil, using a glove made of raw silk instead. Pitta and kapha types should try this as a change from oil. Body-brushing, using a natural bristle brush or a textured mitt, also stimulates lymph circulation, which helps the body rid itself of waste products.

◁ **Use a natural bristle brush for a stimulating body massage while you are bathing.**

Painless detoxification

Spring is traditionally the time for detoxifying. *Swedana*, or sweat therapy, adds to the benefits of massage by helping the body cleanse itself through the pores, while a cleansing diet eases the pressure on digestion, promoting radiantly clear skin and boundless vitality.

steaming

For deep cleaning the skin, steam baths offer an easy solution and the benefits are instantly noticeable. The moist heat allows the pores to open and sweat flushes out impurities. Steam softens the outer layer of skin, encourages renewal by increasing circulation, and helps shed the dead cells – traditionally removed with a metal scraper. For those who can't stand damp heat, or who suffer from an excess of kapha dosha, a sauna may be an effective alternative.

Start with a shower, then oil your skin while still damp, before entering the steam room, to nourish the skin and bring your dosha back into balance. Shower again after steaming, and finish the treatment with a refreshing cool splash: the combination of hot steam and cold pool or shower is profoundly revitalizing.

At home, enjoy the benefits of steam by running a very hot bath and oiling your skin while you relax beside the bath and wait for it to cool. Throw a bag of herbs into the water, choosing a blend to suit your skin or your dosha. When the bath is a comfortable temperature, massage the oil off with an *ubtan*, or herbal powder, then bathe off the residues and finish with a cool shower.

a cleansing diet

Rigorous fasts can cause health problems, including a serious vata or pitta imbalance, but semi-fasting for a few days can help clear accumulated waste. Choose vegetables, fruits and grains that suit your dosha.

• Start the day by drinking a cup of hot water with a dash of fresh lemon juice, and add some honey if you wish.

◁ Oil your skin before a steam bath and shower afterwards, using a massage mitt or sponge to slough off dead skin and leave yourself glowing.

▷ A bath offers two ways to benefit from the effects of hot water. Run it very hot and sit beside it, luxuriating in the steam. When it's cooled enough, step in and relax.

△ **Wake up to the refreshing taste of hot water with a splash of lemon and a trickle of honey.**

• For breakfast, at least half an hour later, squeeze some fresh fruit juice.

• A light lunch should be your main meal, consisting of boiled or steamed vegetables and grains. Eat slowly, so you notice when you're comfortably full.

• In the early evening, drink some fresh vegetable soup or vegetable juice.

• Throughout the day, except within about an hour of your lunch or supper, drink plain hot water or diluted vegetable juice whenever you wish.

If you're following this regime for less than four days, you can cut out the midday grains. Otherwise you can continue for up to 10 days, but no longer, because the diet does not provide all the nutrients you need in the long term.

the secret of eternal youth

Rasayana is Ayurveda's method of staying young. It includes taking herbal remedies selected by a practitioner, practising yoga asanas, and doing *pranayama*, or breathing exercises. Since toxins accelerate the aging process, it also means keeping your intake of these to a minimum.

Eating well becomes more than a question of balancing nutrients: food actually reduces your life force if it's stale, overprocessed, laden with chemicals or irradiated. Alcohol is doubly toxic, through its befuddling influence on the brain as well as its physical effects on the liver.

mental discipline

Ayurveda believes that your health and vitality are strongly influenced by factors such as the environment and your own outlook. Rasayana may require changing your whole lifestyle. How much do you want to keep your energy and your wrinkle-free complexion?

You need to check whether you're producing toxic thoughts. Anger, envy, dishonesty, resentment, greed, callousness and even anxiety can all sap your life force. Just let such feelings go if you can; otherwise seek a practical short-term form of therapy to help root them out. If you spend too much time delving into the reasons for these unworthy thoughts, you're giving them undue attention.

What about your relations with the people around you? Ayurveda values harmony and teaches that you should seek to create it in all areas. If your efforts to free your mind of toxic thoughts are sabotaged by someone who drives you mad, either come to terms with them or keep out of the way. If it's a family member, listen to their grievances and try to understand them.

outside influences

Ensure that your environment isn't dragging you down. Bad air and water are obvious dangers. But do you live in an ugly environment? Can you often hear noisy neighbours or angry car drivers? If you're in the country, are you affected by chemical sprays? Are your surroundings more demoralizing than invigorating? You can build up resistance to outside factors, but it all uses energy that could be better spent.

Your occupation and daily life should tend towards harmony, with the natural world as well as with other people. Is your job worth doing, or does it cause harm? Do you live a wasteful, high-consumption life? Consider whether you need to move house, change jobs or rethink your way of life.

▽ **Oiling the skin is an essential element of Indian beauty, and is also believed to help clear the body of ama, or toxic residues.**

Bringing meditation into your life

Meditation is part of the detoxifying process, helping to clear waste products from the mind. By counteracting stress and promoting a balanced lifestyle, it creates health benefits that show on your face and body. It's simply a way of focusing the mind, freeing up mental energy by stilling the chatter that runs endlessly through our heads. Each time you meditate successfully, your heart slows down, your blood pressure drops and and you move into the relaxed but alert "alpha" state – thinking clearly and living in the moment.

Meditation can increase concentration, aid healing, ease the symptoms of many health conditions, break the habit of worrying and slow the aging process. In rare cases, it can trigger psychological problems – go to your doctor if this happens, since it may have revealed a disorder needing treatment. Also check with your doctor before starting meditation if you have any medical condition, especially one that affects your heart or blood pressure.

beginning meditation

It's easiest to get into the habit of meditation if you do it at the same time and place every day. Choose one form of meditation (for example, counting breaths) and stick to it for at least a week. Set a timer for 10 minutes once a day and you may notice improvements before the end of the week.

Sit on a comfortable straight-backed chair with your feet on the floor and close your eyes. Straight away, your mind will be filled with chatter. You can't relax, you have a brilliant idea, you've remembered something important. Don't do battle with these distractions. As thoughts enter your mind just let them drift on out. When, inevitably, you realise your mind has wandered, calmly bring it back to the meditation without criticism.

Always keep your back straight to let energy move freely. Keep your breathing steady and remain aware of it throughout.

△ **A candle flame can be an aid to meditation – a simple, calming point on which to focus while your mind comes gently to rest.**

counting breaths

Let your breathing slow down, then count each breath just before you take a new one. In-out, one. In-out, two. In-out, three. Count up to 10, then start again. Before long your breath becomes steady and it becomes easier to bring your focus back after each detour. You stop fidgeting and begin to feel a sense of peace.

mantra meditation

A classic form of ayurvedic meditation is repeating a sacred sound, or mantra, over and over again, keeping your attention on the sound. Or you can repeat a word of phrase you find helpful, such as "Om" or "Stillness" or "I am calm". Try to feel nothing but that quality filling you.

▷ **In the Western world, we feel we have to keep busy. Ayurveda, with its concept of balance in all things, reminds us of the value of stillness too.**

◁ Most cultures have developed techniques to still the mind: another traditional method is prayer. Both individuals and society can benefit from rediscovering a peaceful space.

sound and movement, you may be motivated by chanting mantras and walking meditation. If your dosha is aggravated, choose a slow and soothing method. Do try to practise seated meditation, because this is a powerful calming and centring force.

Pitta dosha gives you the drive to succeed at whatever you take up. You can benefit from all kinds of meditation, working on emptying your mind. Any obsessive thoughts soon make themselves obvious by clinging on there. Don't give them attention at all – just quietly waft them away. Mindfulness meditation is also ideal, giving you something else to occupy that space. Since you love beauty and colour, you could try meditating on a mandala, a flame or a favourite flower.

Since kapha people are naturally quiet and calm, you don't need to work on stillness. Instead, try working on keeping the mind focused. Physical activity is always useful for kapha dosha, so you may get more benefit from a moving meditation. Try the livelier forms, such as dancing.

▽ Just one session of meditation can leave you feeling better, and long-term practice can transform your life.

mandala meditation

Gaze at one of these beautiful, complex paintings and let yourself feel the devotion that went into creating it. Keep your focus on the mandala itself, letting any thoughts it inspires drift away. Go on blinking naturally.

candle meditation

This peaceful method is ideal for times when you feel upset. Focus on the beautiful flame, without letting your imagination take over. Just be in this moment, looking at this flame. Remember to blink frequently so your eyes don't become sore.

moving meditation

Movement prevents the restlessness that stops some people meditating. A simple method is walking slowly, regulating your steps to the slow rhythm of your breath. Meditative exercises such as yoga and t'ai chi are also effective.

Experienced meditators can bring the same mental focus to their activities. The key is to do something just complex enough to engage your mind without taking an effort of concentration, while remaining aware of your steady breathing. A steady, rhythmic movement is most helpful, as in swimming. Dancing is uplifting – even though your breathing speeds up, the music and joyful movements can successfully flip you into the alpha state.

mindfulness

A different route to the alpha state is mindfulness meditation, when instead of trying to switch off you focus fully on what you're doing. When you're massaging yourself, for example, instead of planning or day-dreaming, just be totally aware of the fragrance of the oil, the feel of your skin on different parts of the body, the nurturing movements of your hands.

meditation for your dosha

Vata energy is rather speedy, so if you have a predominance of this you'll gain a lot from the calming effects of meditation. Being sensitive to subtle energy and attracted to

The colour of energy

According to Ayurvedic philosophy, colours have healing or harmful properties that can affect our bodies as well as our moods. Each shade contains different wavelengths of light energy, and generates different vibrations that subtly affect our own energies. The body's seven important energy centres, the chakras, are depicted in the form of many-petalled lotuses or whirling wheels of colour. These centres draw in energy from the universe and supply it to our physical and non-physical bodies. The energy channel that connects all the chakras follows the course of the spine.

using colour

The effect of colour is recognized by many people who don't care about the theories but just do what works: they paint fast-food eateries bright red – to make us eat up and leave quickly – and hospitals in healing blues and greens. We are acknowledging the power of colour when we see red, feel blue, lapse into a brown study or walk around under our own personal grey cloud.

Like everything else, shades of colour have *gunas*, or inner qualities. You can train your eye to pick out those that are sattvic: their clear tones promote harmony and

▷ **Green is an ideal colour to use for a workplace, as it balances *tejas* – the mental fire that fuels intellectual efforts – and promotes a feeling of calm alertness.**

enlightenment. Harsh, over-bright rajasic hues put your nerves on edge, and muddy tamasic shades dull the senses.

Though we can't always control the colours that surround us, we can choose what to wear and how to decorate our

▽ **If you're run down or lethargic, surround yourself with energizing colours and feel them gently raise your spirits.**

homes. An insomniac whose bedroom is red or orange, for example, would be well advised to redecorate in a gentle shade of blue. If you sometimes feel out of touch with reality, repaint any white walls with warm pastels. Sombre colours (including certain cold shades of blue) can deepen depression. A clear violet will help you to pray or meditate, and green will keep your judgement unclouded while you work.

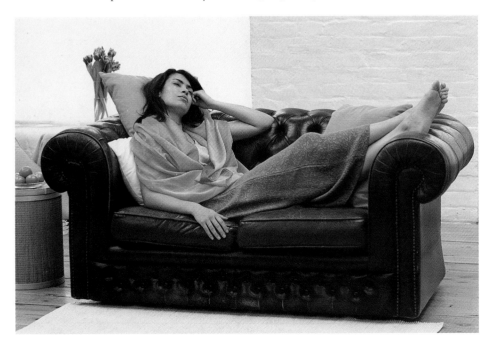

COLOURS FOR BALANCE

When your dominant dosha is aggravated, you can choose colours that help bring it back into balance.

Vata needs warming and grounding with colours such as red, orange or yellow. Avoid violet or purple, which can make vata types light-headed. Pastel shades such as pink are often helpful.

Pitta needs cooling colours such as blue, violet or white. Avoid red, orange, yellow, black, and rajasic shades of any colour.

Kapha needs warm, bright, energizing colours such as red, orange, yellow or violet. Avoid brown or grey.

▷ Warm colours have a nourishing, grounding effect on light-headed vata, and can help create a state of relaxed alertness. These rich shades ease feelings of coldness and dryness.

the chakras

Ayurveda teaches that each chakra governs a different part of the body and supplies a distinctive kind of energy. A blockage in one of the chakras will cause specific diseases or emotional disorders. If you feel that you have a problem in one of these areas, try visualizing the chakra bathed in light of its own colour while meditating.

Muladhara, the root chakra: The first chakra is situated just behind the genitals. Its colour is red, and it is the source of strength and stability. The first chakra governs the body's eliminatory systems and its influence makes you practical and grounded. When it

is blocked or damaged in some way you may suffer from lower back pain, or become angry or disorganized.

Svadisthana, the sacral chakra: The second chakra is orange and lies just below the navel. It inspires passion, sexuality and creativity. It governs the reproductive system. Potential problems include sexual problems, self-pity and cystitis.

Manipura, the solar plexus chakra: The third chakra is yellow and provides willpower. It rules the digestive system and many internal organs. Problems include fear, low self-esteem and digestive disorders.

Anahata, the heart chakra: The fourth chakra is green and it is the source of compassion and equilibrium. Its area of influence is the heart and blood circulation. Problems include despair, unbalanced judgement, heart and lung disorders.

Vishudda, the throat chakra: The fifth chakra is blue. It rules the mouth and the thyroid gland, and the ability to learn. Problems include sore throats and difficulty in speaking out.

Ajna, the brow chakra: The sixth chakra, or third eye, is indigo. Situated in the middle of the forehead, it is the source of intuition and governs the nervous system and pituitary gland. It is the spot we instinctively touch when trying to think. Problems are nightmares, lack of concentration or detachment from reality.

Sahasrara, the crown chakra: The seventh chakra rules the pineal gland and is the source of enlightenment. It is shown coloured either violet or white – which contains all colours. If the crown chakra is blocked you may feel confused, or behave selfishly and unethically.

▽ Tranquil shades of blue and clean, clear white help keep pitta cool on even the hottest days.

◁ The chakras act as gateways or energy centres, drawing in energy from the universe and distributing it to our physical and non-physical bodies.

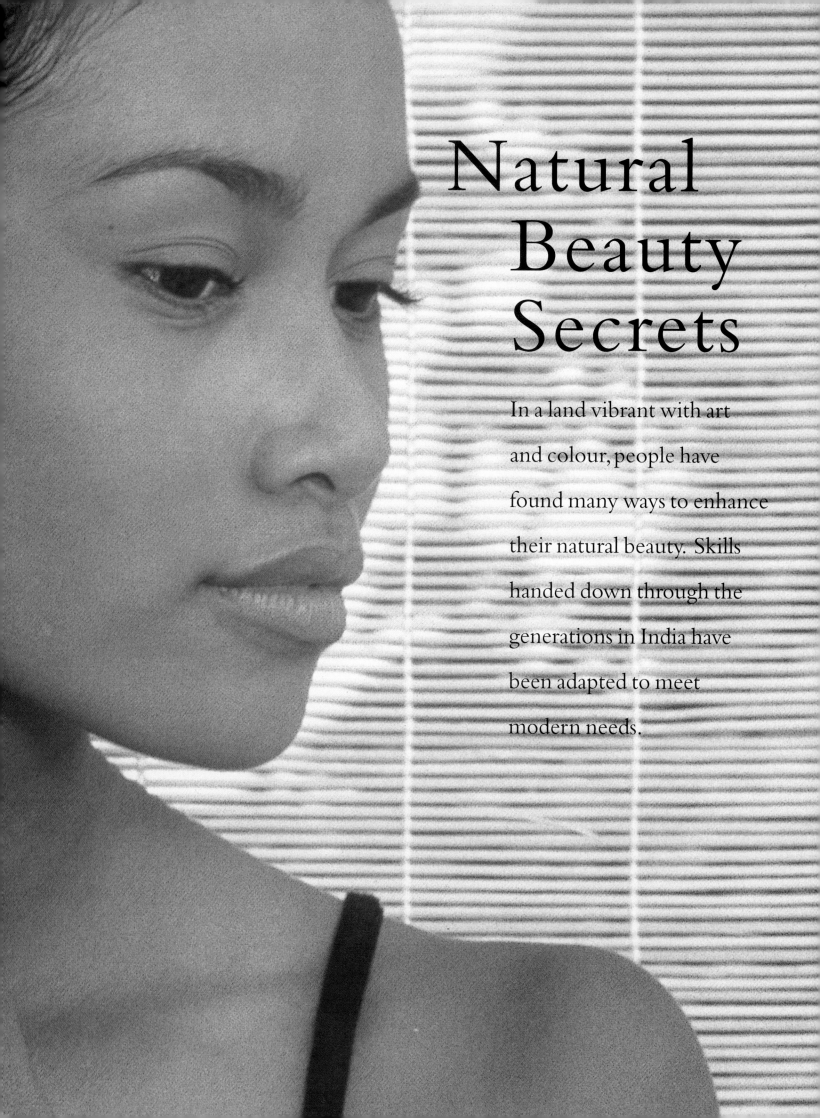

Natural Beauty Secrets

In a land vibrant with art and colour, people have found many ways to enhance their natural beauty. Skills handed down through the generations in India have been adapted to meet modern needs.

A home facial

Ayurvedic beauty treatments don't just improve skin quality: they're also an antidote to stress. The full routine for a facial treatment takes about an hour, so dedicate one evening every week or month to treat yourself luxuriously, but you can use the cleansing, toning and (for dry skins) moisturizing steps of this facial every day. Commercially made Ayurvedic beauty products are internationally available, but for those who like to make their own, recipes for each stage of the treatment are given on the following pages.

cleansing with oil

Oil is a good make-up remover for all skin types, and is ideal for cleansing off city grime or dust. You can make up your own blend, using a suitable base oil for your skin type, or use a base oil alone. Apply oil with your fingertips in a circular motion. Instead of washing the oil off, Indian women traditionally blot it up with a herbal powder called an *ubtan*.

ubtans

These powders clean and stimulate the skin, and can be used as a cleanser alone or after applying oil. The simplest ubtan is a mix of plain besan (chickpea or gram flour) made into a paste with a few drops of liquid: use lemon juice for oily skin or warm milk for dry skin. The paste should be firm and not too liquid. Apply to the skin with the fingertips using circular or upward movements, and when it feels dry massage it off with warm water.

More complex mixtures, containing herbs and grains, are used as exfoliants, usually after a herbal heat treatment. For skin that's not blemished or sensitive, it's a good idea to use a slightly coarser formulation every few weeks, always avoiding the delicate eye area. If your skin is sensitive, though, ensure the ubtan is finely ground – and resist that enthusiastic pitta tendency to scrub too hard.

▷ **Oil is excellent for removing make-up and nourishing all types of skin. It enters the finest pores without causing harm. Almond oil, rich in Vitamin E, is the traditional favourite**.

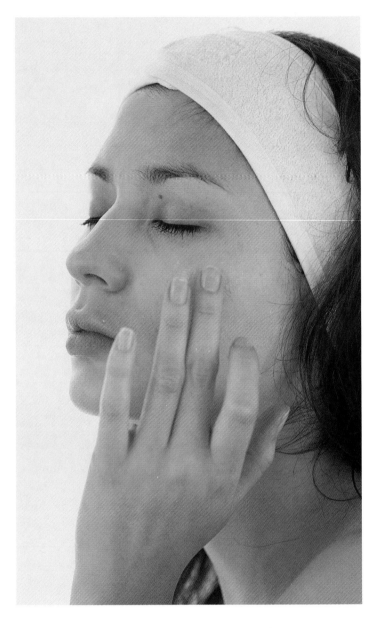

herbal heat treatment

A weekly heat treatment suits most skin types, though once a month is enough for dry and mature skins. Damp heat opens the pores, encourages sweat to flush out ingrained dirt and brings oxygen-rich blood to renew the skin. You may choose to put oil on your skin first, since the heat helps the oil penetrate more deeply. But don't leave cleansing oil on, or you'll be drawing dirt back into the skin.

Herbal steam: Sit with your head forward over a bowl of hot, herb-infused water, draped in a towel to stop the steam escaping, for about 5 minutes. Stop immediately if you feel dizzy or overheated.

Herbal compress: Soak several face cloths in hot, herb-infused water, and wring out. Sitting with your head back and supported, put the cloths over your face and relax for 5 minutes. As the cloths cool down, wring them out in the hot water again.

Herbal bath: Infuse a bag of herbs in your bath and let the heat open your pores.

Finish by patting your face with a clean cloth wrung out in cool water. Give your face a cooling splash of toner or water, then rest for a few minutes to cool down.

▷ Any nourishing or rejuvenating facial treatment, such as an oil massage, should work upwards from below your collarbones – an area that is all too often neglected.

oil massage

This is a traditional Indian technique. Oils are highly prized in Ayurveda, and considered essential to the healthy functioning of the body, but moisturizer can be used instead of oil if you prefer.

Warm some oil and pour a little into your hands. Starting just below your collarbones, smooth it into your skin using long strokes upwards and outwards, or clockwise circular movements. Continue for up to 10 minutes, covering your throat and face. Your touch should be just firm enough to move the skin slightly, without dragging it. Be especially careful not to drag dry or mature skin. Those with kapha skin should wipe off the oil before continuing.

facepack or mask

Few treatments give your skin such a quick lift as a facepack. These simple treatments, based on fruit or vegetables, can be left on for up to an hour, while you have a massage or meditate (you may need to be lying down if the mask is runny; try the Corpse yoga

▽ Take a break while the mask does its work – use the time for some other pampering treat.

pose). A mask is a stronger version of a facepack, using a powder such as flour or clay to penetrate the pores more deeply. It should be left on for 10–20 minutes.

To remove the facepack or mask, dab it with water (for oily skin) or milk (for dry skin) to soften it, then gently massage and rinse the mix off your skin.

toning

Remove any residues and soothe the skin with a splash of cool flower water or, for oily skin, witch hazel and flower water. Skin that

is very oily or has darker patches can be rubbed with a slice of lemon and left for a few minutes before rinsing off.

moisturizing

Only moisturize skin that feels dry. If you have oily skin or acne and follow the Ayurvedic process, you needn't use a moisturizer – none of the cleansing recipes will strip the skin of oil.

▽ A slice of lemon helps lighten darker patches, but don't use this on dry or sensitive skin.

First step: cleansing

Traditional wisdom is a dynamic resource, adapting to new conditions as it passes down through the generations. Indian families who move to other countries often modify their age-old recipes to suit what they have to hand, replacing ingredients that are hard to find outside India with others that are easily obtainable, including essential oils.

You can turn your kitchen cupboard into a beauty treasure-trove, as practically all the ingredients needed for the following recipes are used in everyday Indian cookery. All are available from Asian stores, and most can be found in supermarkets.

▷ Ingredients for an ubtan (clockwise from front): ground coriander, liquorice sticks, besan, ground cumin and ground fenugreek.

△ Oils to suit your skin, from left: almond for all complexions, sesame for dry, sunflower for oily.

cleansing cream

The best oils for cleansing are almond, sesame and sunflower. Alternatively, you can use this light cream cleanser.

ingredients
- 7.5 ml/½ tbsp beeswax
- 30 ml/2 tbsp coconut oil
- 30 ml/2 tbsp almond oil
- 60 ml/4 tbsp cucumber juice (or water)
- 1.5 ml/¼ tsp borax
- 15 ml/1 tbsp witch hazel
- few drops rose water

ALLERGY ALERT

Before applying any cosmetic to your face, test it on your inner arm, leaving it for as long as you intend to leave it on your face. If any redness or irritation develops, wash off the mixture at once and discard it.

Melt the beeswax in a non-metallic bowl over a pan of hot water, and add the oils. In a separate bowl, heat the cucumber juice and borax (a good natural emulsifier) until the borax is completely dissolved. Add the witch hazel and remove from the heat. Combine the contents of the two bowls and allow to cool a little, then add the rose water. Beat the mixture until it cools and thickens.

herbal ubtan

This a traditional Indian cleanser. Many different blends are possible, but all have gentle softening and cleansing effects.

ingredients
- ground coriander
- ground cumin
- ground fenugreek
- ground liquorice
- besan (chickpea flour)

Mix together equal quantities of all of the ingredients and then store your mixed powder in a clean and airtight container. You will need about a small handful for one treatment. The dry base blend should be mixed to a paste consistency with the appropriate liquid ingredient for immediate use whenever it is needed.

- For oily, combination or blemished skin, mix the base blend to a paste with yogurt or diluted lemon juice.
- For dry or mature skin, mix the ubtan with milk or cream.
- For normal skin, or if the other combinations feel too sticky, mix with water or rose water.

Mix to a smooth, soft paste, then rub it into your skin – gently for dry vata or sensitive pitta complexions – using small circular movements. Massage off with warm, followed by cool, water.

△ If you've made more than you need for a facial, why not give your feet and legs a treat too?

◁ **Orange peel contains astringent oils that cleanse away excessive skin secretions and help to remove blemishes caused by blocked pores.**

almond ubtan

This mixture is especially useful for reducing a pitta or vata imbalance, or for dry or sensitive skin.

ingredients
- walnuts
- fine oatmeal
- ground almonds

Grind the walnuts to a coarse powder and mix with equal quantities of the oatmeal and ground almonds. Store the mixture in an airtight container. To use, mix a small handful of the powder to a paste using water (for oily skin) or milk (for dry skin).

▽ **Preparing ingredients, such as these walnuts for an ubtan for dry skin, is part of an almost meditative process of self-nourishment.**

orange peel ubtan

This is useful for people with oily skin or a kapha imbalance, who should use it every second day. It helps remove blackheads gently and leaves skin feeling smooth. Start off by using equal quantities of all the ingredients. Later, you may decide to vary the proportions to suit your own skin.

ingredients
- lentils
- wheat
- dried orange peel
- fine oatmeal
- besan (chickpea flour)

Grind the lentils, wheat and dried orange peel to a coarse powder. For sensitive pitta skin, grind the powders more finely. Mix all the ingredients together and store the blend in an airtight container.

MILK AND SUGAR

These make the simplest facial. Moisten your face with water, then gently massage clean with a teaspoonful of sugar. Tone with a splash of water. Moisturize with skin from the top of boiled milk that's been left to cool. Leave this on for 2 minutes, then massage off with water.

To use the ubtan, mix a small handful of the powder to a soft paste using a few drops of water, or lemon juice, or both, depending on your skin type. Use the paste as a facial scrub.

The next steps: heat and oil

For body massage, Ayurvedic practitioners normally choose an oil that will help to bring the doshas into balance, such as sesame oil to reduce vata or kapha and coconut oil to cool an excess of pitta. For the face and throat, however, they base their choice on skin type and condition – which are often an expression of dosha energy anyway.

In general, vata energy is expressed in dry skin, pitta in sensitive skin and kapha in oily skin. So you may wish to use treatments that suit your skin condition, while eating and following other guidelines to pacify the relevant dosha.

skin types

Classic vata skin is thin and fine-pored, dry, cool and often dark. This fragile complexion needs very gentle care and moisturizing. It should never be rubbed hard or dragged.

▽ **For an easy steam treatment, pour a few drops of herbal oil blend into the bath and relax.**

Pitta skin is soft, warm and rosy, but often sensitive. Avoid harsh chemicals or anything that could cause a rash or inflammation. Pittas often have combination skin, with an oily T-zone of forehead, nose and chin but drier skin on the cheeks and beside the mouth. Common problems are acne and patches of pigmentation.

Kapha skin is strong, thick and naturally moist. It's therefore slow to show signs of aging or environmental damage, but it is prone to enlarged pores, blackheads and excessive oiliness.

If, like most people, you are influenced by two doshas, you should note which one seems dominant in your complexion. You may be mainly kapha, but if your skin is sensitive to heat and chemicals, and is much drier on your cheeks and beside your mouth, it's expressing pitta energy and needs to be treated for this. Your skin condition will also vary with external factors such as the weather: the cold dryness of winter increases vata energy, for example, and may affect your skin accordingly.

herbal steam treatment

Add a scented mixture of herbs and spices to hot water for a gentle heat treatment. Test the steam with your inner arm before allowing it near your face.

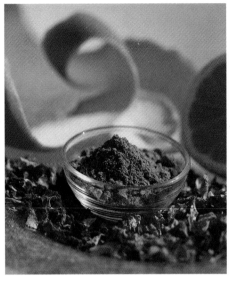

△ **Fresh ingredients boiled in water release their fragrance and healing powers in steam.**

ingredients
- half a lemon
- strips of orange peel
- pinch of pure sandalwood powder
- dried rose petals

Possible added ingredients you could use:
- For oily skin: liquorice root, lavender, fennel seeds, rosemary.
- For mature skin: liquorice root, fennel seeds, clove, grated ginger, mint.
- For dry skin: liquorice root, bay leaf, chamomile.
- For blemished skin: liquorice root, lemon grass, lavender, dandelion root.
- For normal skin: liquorice root, thyme, chamomile, fennel seeds, lavender.

Put at least 1.2 litres/2 pints/5 cups water in an enamelled or non-metallic pan and add the lemon and about two handfuls of a mixture of the remaining ingredients. Cover and bring to the boil, stirring occasionally, then remove from the heat. Leave covered and allow to cool until the steam is a comfortable temperature.

◁ **If you're short of time – or herbs – even plain hot water can be used to steam oiled skin.**

△ **Sesame or almond oil, infused with jasmine, makes a soothing massage oil for dry skin.**

facial massage oils

The base oils can be used alone, but do try making a herbal oil for face or body massage: two methods are given below. Some infused oils can be bought ready-made, or you could add a drop of essential oil. (A few essential oils should be avoided in pregnancy; check with an expert before using.)

simple herbal oil

ingredients

- handful of fresh herb (see box)
- 250 ml/8 fl oz/1 cup base oil (see box)

Crush the herb leaves using a pestle and mortar, then add a small amount of your

HERBAL OILS FOR YOUR SKIN TYPE

- Normal skin: almond oil with lavender or geranium.
- Skin infections: almond oil with neem, sandalwood or triphala.
- Rough or dehydrated skin: almond oil with rose, manjishtha or arjun.
- Dry skin: almond or sesame oil with rose or jasmine.
- Mature skin: almond or sesame oil with lavender or frankincense.
- Oily skin: almond, sunflower or jojoba oil with lemon or bergamot.
- Blemished skin: almond, sunflower or jojoba oil with lavender or tea tree.
- Cellulite: almond oil with lemon or orange.

chosen base oil and blend thoroughly. Now add this blend to the rest of the oil, pour into a screw-top jar and shake well. Keep in a cool, dark place and shake several times a day for three days before using.

herbal oil infusion

ingredients

- 4 parts base oil (see box)
- 16 parts water
- 1 part ground or powdered herb (see box)

Measure the oil into an enamelled or non-metallic pan and add the water and your chosen herb. Bring to the boil over a medium heat, stirring briskly, then reduce the heat and leave to simmer gently, stirring occasionally, until all of the water has evaporated. Depending on the amount of infused oil you are making, this may take an hour or more. You could leave the pan on the back burner while you are preparing food, unless you are cooking something with a strong smell that could affect the oil.

▽ **Rosemary adds a clean, sharp tang to a herbal steam for oily or teenage skin.**

RULES OF THUMB

Traditionally, people learnt these recipes by watching their mothers and aunts preparing them. They were tailored to each person's needs, so would vary according to their individual constitution, their current state of health and the season. Ingredients would be measured in handfuls, and the proportions given here are guides rather than rules: experiment to find, or create, a formulation that suits you.

△ **So precious it was once a gift for kings, frankincense makes a nourishing blend for mature skin.**

Deep-cleansing facepacks and masks

△ **Masks contain earth or flour, so don't apply near the delicate eye area or leave them on for more than 20 minutes, as they can be drying.**

Applying the very simplest cleansing and nourishing facepacks involves little more than squashing ripe fruit on to your face. Most fruits and vegetables can be used in this way, though harder types need to be grated or puréed: experiment with the suggestions given here to find what produces the best result on your skin. Smooth the facepack on with your fingers – or, if you find it easier, paint it on with a pastry brush kept for this purpose – and leave it on your face for up to 20 minutes (unless stated otherwise) while you relax. At the end of that time, massage the facepack off your skin and then finish by rinsing with water.

Clay, oatmeal or besan (chickpea or gram flour) can be added to any of the facepack recipes to make a mask that aids the cleansing process by drawing out dirt from deep in the pores. Oat flour is very soothing for eczema, while chickpea flour can leave skin feeling very taut, so is best combined with other dry ingredients. Mix the mask to a consistency that won't slide straight off your face – experiment on the back of your hand – and leave for up to 20 minutes before massaging and rinsing it off.

simple facepack

ingredients

• selection of fruit and/or vegetables (see box)
• 5 ml/1 tsp yogurt or almond oil

In a non-metallic bowl, chop, grate or mash the fruit and vegetables to a pulp. Strain off the excess juice for a healthy drink, and add the yogurt (for oily skin) or oil (for dry skin) to the pulp. Spread or brush the mixture over your face and neck, avoiding the delicate skin around the eyes. Lie down for at least 10 minutes while it takes effect, then massage and rinse off with cool water.

skin rejuvenator

This is kind to mature skin and can help reduce the appearance of wrinkles.

ingredients

• handful of fresh scented geranium (*Pelargonium graveolens*) leaves
• rose water to cover

Soak the geranium leaves in rose water for a few hours until softened, then spread on your face and lie down for 15–30 minutes.

avocado facepack

Egg white and lemon juice usually suit oily complexions, but the addition of avocado, rich in natural oils, makes this a great soother for dry skin too.

ingredients

• 1 avocado
• 5 ml/1 tsp lemon juice
• 1 egg white

Mash the avocado, mix in the other ingredients and apply to the face.

△ **Experiment to find what suits you: the richness of avocado makes a soothing facepack.**

apple facepack

This suits all skin types. If you have very oily skin, you may wish to use jojoba oil instead of almond.

FACEPACK INGREDIENTS FOR YOUR SKIN TYPE

Sharp-tasting fruits, such as grape, lemon, tomato or peach, should be combined with a more soothing, starchy fruit or vegetable, such as banana. Be careful if you include grape in a mixture, as it has a peeling effect on the skin; don't use it at all if your skin is dry or sensitive.

• Normal skin: avocado, banana, courgette, grape, peach.
• Dry skin: avocado, banana, carrot, melon, pear.
• Oily or combination skin: cabbage, cucumber, lemon, pear, strawberries, tomatoes, tangerine.
• Mature skin: apple, avocado, banana.
• Blemished skin: apple, cabbage, plums (boiled and allowed to cool), tomato.
• In hot weather: cucumber, strawberries.

△ **Relax while an apple facepack rebalances your skin and cucumber reduces any puffiness.**

ingredients

- ½ small apple, peeled and grated
- 15 ml/1 tbsp honey
- 1 egg yolk
- 15 ml/1 tbsp cider or wine vinegar
- 45 ml/3 tbsp almond oil

Mix together all ingredients.

spot remedy facepack

ingredients

- 1 egg white
- 5 ml/1 tsp honey
- 5 ml/1 tsp carrot juice
- 5 ml/1 tsp crushed garlic

Beat the egg white until stiff. Mix in the other ingredients and apply for 20 minutes to help heal spots and blemishes.

honey and egg facepack

This instantly rejuvenates dry skin.

ingredients

- 2.5 ml/½ tsp honey
- 1 egg yolk
- 15 ml/1 tbsp dried skimmed milk

Mix to a paste and leave on for 20 minutes.

juicy mask

Yogurt cleanses the skin, while the juices feed it with vitamins and minerals.

ingredients

- 15 ml/1 tbsp powdered brewer's yeast
- 2.5 ml/½ tsp yogurt
- 5 ml/1 tsp orange juice
- 5 ml/1 tsp carrot juice
- 5 ml/1 tsp almond oil

Mix all the ingredients into a paste. If you have oily skin or darker patches, add 5 ml/1 tsp lemon juice; for very dry skin, double the oil content.

clarifying mask

ingredients

- 10 ml/2 tsp ground almonds
- 5 ml/1 tsp rose water
- 2.5 ml/½ tsp honey

Mix into a paste and apply as a thin layer. Rinse off with cool rose water.

△ **Add a little light oil, such as almond or jojoba, to counteract the drying effect of face masks on delicate vata skin.**

oatmeal mask

Use yogurt to bind the dry ingredients if you have oily skin, or almond oil for dry skin. For other skin types, choose whichever you prefer – try one version on each cheek and see which feels better.

ingredients

- 10 ml/2 tsp fine oatmeal
- 30 ml/2 tbsp powdered orange peel
- yogurt or almond oil

Mix the oatmeal and powdered orange peel together and add enough yogurt or almond oil to make a paste.

potato mask

Rich in Vitamin C, potatoes also tighten the skin, making this a good choice for tired or mature complexions.

ingredients

- 15 ml/1 tbsp potato juice
- 15 ml/1 tbsp multani mitti (fuller's earth)

Mix together thoroughly to make a paste and spread on the skin.

BESAN (CHICKPEA FLOUR) MASKS
- For oily skin: mix besan with some olive oil and lemon juice.
- For dry or normal skin: mix besan with some olive oil and yogurt.

spot remedy mask

This is effective against spots and blemishes.

ingredients

- 1 egg yolk
- 15 ml/1 tbsp powdered brewer's yeast
- 15 ml/1 tbsp sunflower oil

Mix to a paste and apply to the face. After 15 minutes rinse off with milk.

orange mask

This is suitable for dry skin.

ingredients

- 5 ml/1 tsp freshly squeezed orange juice
- 15 ml/1 tbsp multani mitti (fuller's earth)
- 15 ml/1 tbsp rose water
- 15 ml/1 tbsp liquid honey

Mix all the ingredients together to make a paste and smooth lightly on to the skin.

EGG ON YOUR FACE
When you need to look good and haven't time for a full treatment, just try an egg. For oily skin, beat an egg white and spread on to your face. Leave to dry and then wash off thoroughly. This tightens skin for a temporary face-lifting effect. If you have dry skin, use the whole egg, beaten. You can also use egg white or whole egg, depending on your skin type, as a substitute for oil or yogurt in herbal ubtans and facepacks.

△ **Egg feeds the skin and binds powders.**

toning and moisturizing

A splash of cool filtered or spring water refreshes skin after any treatment. Flower waters add their own natural benefits, and gently close pores without the harshness of alcohol-based toners. For oily skin, try water with a dash of vinegar, or rose water with a dash of witch hazel.

flower waters

Rose water is perfect for skin care. Mildly astringent, it soothes and rehydrates skin. It's cooling in a hot climate, reduces inflammation, and the subtle fragrance is said to have antidepressant and aphrodisiac qualities. Buy the highest quality you can find, or make your own.

Rose water makes a refreshing spray, especially in the dryness of air-conditioned rooms or the stuffy heat of a plane, and also helps to set make-up. A cloth or cotton pads wrung out in rose water and placed over closed eyes is the kindest treatment when your eyes are sore.

Other flowers can be used in the same way. Lavender water has long been prized for its cleansing, deodorant properties and refreshing scent. In hot weather it is ideal to use over the entire body – and also for spraying on clothes and bedlinen.

▽ **Simple pleasure: a splash of plain water revitalizes your mind and refreshes your skin.**

rose water

Use equal quantities, by volume, of rose petals and pure water to give a delicately scented result. Increase the water's strength by using more petals, as long as the water still covers them. For an even stronger scent, use dried rose petals: simply shake fresh petals into a paper bag, loosely close the top, hang up and leave to dry.

ingredients

- 1 cup fresh scented rose petals, tightly packed
- 1 cup spring or filtered water

Put the petals in a heatproof, non-metallic container. Boil the water and pour it over the petals. Cover and leave to cool. Decant into a screwtop bottle or jar and store in the fridge.

rose water astringent

For oily or blemished skin.

ingredients

- 1 part rose water
- 1 part witch hazel

Pour both ingredients into a screwtop jar or bottle and shake to mix.

△ **The fragrance of rose water has been treasured throughout history.**

rose water soother

A treat for a dry complexion and tired skin under the eyes.

ingredients

- 250 ml/8 fl oz/1 cup rose water
- 1 drop sandalwood oil
- 1 drop rose, tea rose or rose geranium essential oil

Pour all ingredients into a screwtop jar or bottle and shake to mix.

lavender water

ingredients

- handful of fresh lavender heads, stems removed
- 475 ml/16 fl oz/2 cups filtered or spring water

Put the flowers into a jar with a screw top and pour the water over them. Leave for a day, shaking occasionally. For a stronger scent, leave it for up to three weeks, taking the top off every few days to check the scent. Strain off the water into a clean jar or bottle and keep in the refrigerator.

flower water refresher

ingredients

- 1 part water
- 1 part rose water or lavender water
- 2 slices cucumber
- few drops lemon juice (optional, for oily skin)

Combine the water and flower water and refrigerate for 5 minutes. Dip the cucumber slices in the liquid and put over closed eyes while you rest. Pour the remaining liquid into a spray bottle, adding a few drops of lemon juice if you have oily skin. Use as a refreshing spritz for face and throat.

moisturizing cream

Adjust the measurements given to find a consistency that suits your skin, and choose a herbal powder to balance your dosha: white sandalwood or jasmine for pitta, manjishtha for vata, or neem for kapha.

ingredients

- 30 ml/2 tbsp beeswax
- 175 ml/6 fl oz/³/₄ cup almond oil
- pinch of herbal powder (see above) or a few drops rose or jasmine essential oil

Melt the beeswax gently in a non-metallic bowl over hot water. Stir in the oil. Add the herbal powder or essential oil, and whisk until the mixture is soft. Allow to cool.

▷ For a subtle and unique fragrance, look around your garden and pick your favourite blooms to create flower water recipes of your own.

TAKE CARE OF YOURSELF

Don't hurry while giving yourself a facial. If time is short, it's better to leave out some of the steps than to rush through them. As far as possible, ensure that your surroundings are quiet and you're not interrupted. The results can be seen as stress dissolves from your face.

Preparation, too, should be a meditative process. Focus, one by one, on the colours of the ingredients, their textures as they are mixed together, the different scents as they develop, the small sounds of the spoon against the bowl and the feel of the various mixtures on your skin.

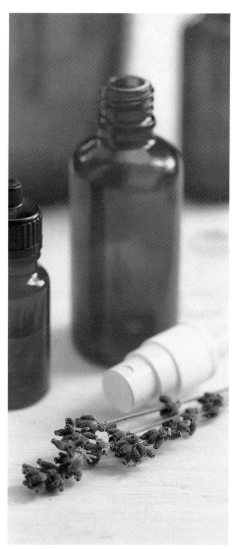

◁ Keep some screwtop jars for mixing and spray bottles for spritzing. Remember to store all natural cosmetics – and even bottled water, once it's opened – in the refrigerator for safety.

SAFE STORAGE

Traditionally, women grew their own plants or bought them freshly picked. They ground their own spices, grains and other powders, and used them immediately, whether in cooking or on their skin. Not many of us have a chance to do the same now, so we need to store ingredients safely.

Dry ingredients should be kept in clean, airtight containers. Stored in a dark cupboard, they should keep their fragrance and potency for weeks or months. Anything moist should be refrigerated to prevent the growth of moulds or bacteria. Since home-made cosmetics don't contain strong preservatives, mix them as you need them and don't keep the leftovers for more than a few days.

An Ayurvedic facelift

Your skin type, build and dosha will determine whether lines or sagging will be more of a problem as your skin ages. Generally, if you're thin and have dry skin you're more likely to develop wrinkles, a problem that besets many vata people. Kaphas are more likely to have oily skin and put on weight. This can bring beauty benefits, but the downside is that extra flesh starts to sag, causing a jowly effect. Anyone ruled by pitta or (like most of us) by more than one dosha could encounter any of these problems. So the best treatment aims to keep them all at bay.

Marma-point facial massage

A 30-minute daily marma-point massage will slow down the effects of time on your face. In Ayurvedic terms you're encouraging the movement of prana, the life force; Western science explains it as releasing muscle stiffness and increasing blood circulation. Sit with your back straight but not arched. It's useful to have a table to lean your elbows on, and to use a mirror to check the positions of your fingers, but close your eyes when you don't need to look. Before starting, massage your shoulders, neck and head for a few minutes: tension in these neighbouring muscles creates tension in your face.

VARYING PRESSURE

Throughout the massage you can either continue the 7–5–7–5–7–5 pressure used in step 1, or simply press once for a count of 7. Either way, press slowly and firmly, pressing inwards against the bone, not upwards or downwards unless specified. You can also vary the direct touch with small circling movements, maintaining the pressure and moving the skin over the bone.

◁ **1** Begin by working on the Third Eye point, slightly above the bridge of your nose. Feel for a slight indentation, which is often the sign of an important marma point. Apply firm pressure for a count of 7 as you breathe out, then reduce to light pressure for 5, breathing in. Repeat 3 times.

◁ **2** Find the point in each eyebrow directly above the centre of the eye, and visualize a line from there up into your hair. Following this line, press your ring finger into the eyebrow point, the index finger into the hairline, and the middle finger between them.

△ **3** Feel for the upper edges of the eye sockets and press firmly with the thumbs. Be careful to press the bone, without letting your thumbs slip into your eyes or eye sockets. Lift your thumbs, move them just above the eye sockets and press again, pushing upwards so that your forehead furrows.

△ **4** Place the tips of your index fingers on your cheek bones, with your other fingertips vertically below them under the centre of each eye, and apply firm pressure.

△ **5** Find a point directly below each cheekbone, still in line with the centre of your eyes. Press inwards and upwards into the bottom of the cheekbone.

△ **6** Put the flat of each ring finger on the outer edge of each eye socket, and spread the other fingers out along a diagonal line to the edge of the ear. Press the fingers firmly.

△ **7** Find a point at the outer edge of each nostril and press diagonally inwards with your third fingers, while your index and middle fingers press inwards and upwards below the cheekbones.

△ **8** Bunch all fingertips close together and press along the space between your top lip and your nose – an area containing numerous marma points. Do the same below your lower lip.

△ **9** Press one thumbtip into the centre of your chin.

△ **10** If you like, pour a little oil or cream suitable for your skin type onto your hands. Bring your hands down the centre of your face, barely touching it, until the heels of your hands are under your chin. Now lightly stroke your fingertips out to the side across the cheekbones, without rubbing the fine skin directly beneath the eyes. Then bring the hands, with a firmer stroke, up the sides of the face. Repeat two or three times. Cup your hands over your closed eyes for several breaths.

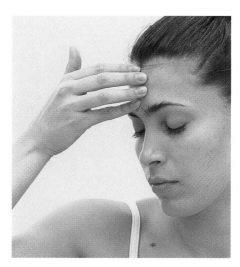

△ **11** Place your fingertips flat on your forehead, then stroke lightly towards the right ear. Repeat on the left. Stroke in both directions several times. If there's any feeling of drag, apply more oil to your skin. Continue the movement into your hair.

◁ **12** Massage your head. Lightly pull sections of hair, making your scalp move in circles over your skull. Finish by combing with your fingers in long movements to the ends of the hair.

When you see the difference a facepack makes to your complexion, why stop there? Indian women have long enjoyed the benefits of herbal pastes, using them to enhance skin quality over the entire body.

Herbal baths are the easiest skincare treatment of all. Simply relax in a warm bath and let the ingredients nourish your skin while the heat eases away tension. Liquid ingredients can be poured straight into the water. Put other ingredients in a muslin bag, swish it around in the bath and leave it in while you soak.

body mask for oily or blemished skin

This mask is designed to detoxify, balance, remove impurities and polish the skin surface, leaving it silky smooth.

ingredients

- 115 g/4 oz/1 cup besan (chickpea flour)
- 5–10 ml/1–2 tsp turmeric
- 30 ml/2 tbsp white sandalwood powder
- 15 ml/1 tbsp red sandalwood powder
- 30 ml/2 tbsp neem leaf powder
- 30 ml/2 tbsp powdered orange peel
- water
- yogurt (optional)

Mix all the dry ingredients together and add water, or a combination of water and yogurt, to make a thin paste. Brush over the skin and leave for about 30 minutes, until dry. Wet the mask with water or milk, then massage off with fairly firm pressure. Rinse with water.

body mask for dry skin

ingredients

- 115 g/4 oz/1 cup besan (chickpea flour)
- 15 ml/1 tbsp white sandalwood powder
- 15 ml/1 tbsp red sandalwood powder
- 15 ml/1 tbsp Indian madder
- 15 ml/1 tbsp arjuna
- 15 ml/1 tbsp brahmi
- 15 ml/1 tbsp shatavari
- unhomogenized milk to mix

△ **Treat your whole body to a revitalizing mask that sloughs off dead cells, letting skin shine.**

Mix the dry ingredients then add the milk, warmed to body temperature, to make a paste. Brush this on to the skin and leave until it is dry. Remove with more of the warm milk.

bridal body mask

This is traditionally used by brides-to-be every day for 10 days before the wedding. It leaves the skin feeling soft and clean. A very simple form can be made using just turmeric and oil.

ingredients

- 15 ml/1 tbsp powdered orange peel
- 15 ml/1 tbsp powdered lemon peel
- 30 ml/2 tbsp ground almonds
- pinch of salt
- 25 g/1 oz/4 tbsp finely ground wheatgerm
- 15 ml/1 tbsp ground thyme
- 7.5 ml/1/2 tbsp turmeric
- almond oil to mix
- few drops jasmine or rose essential oil

Mix all the dry ingredients and add enough almond oil to make a paste. Add the jasmine or rose oil. Spread over the body and leave for 15–20 minutes. Rub off firmly, as though you are gently "sanding" the skin.

QUICK BEAUTY TIP
For the simplest body scrub of all, massage sea salt on to damp skin and shower off.

soothing bath mix

Add to the bath water to calm irritated skin, but don't use this on broken skin.

ingredients

- 120 ml/4 fl oz/1/2 cup cider or wine vinegar
- 30 ml/2 tbsp honey
- 120 ml/4 fl oz/1/2 cup lemon juice
  (or 115 g/4 oz/1 cup oatmeal)

If the sensitivity is intense, leave out the lemon juice as it will sting, and substitute a muslin bag of oatmeal.

▽ **A bath treatment to soften your skin can be as simple as a bagful of plain oatmeal swirled in the water.**

▷ Having your eyebrows professionally threaded gives long-lasting shape and definition, and you can learn to do it yourself.

◁ Time to relax and let the tension drift out of tired muscles. Finishing with a cool shower gives skin a healthy glow.

skin softening bath mix

A very nourishing, soothing combination.

ingredients
- 45 ml/3 tbsp oatmeal
- 15 ml/1 tbsp bran
- 15 ml/1 tbsp ground almonds
- 15 ml/1 tbsp wheat flour
- few drops rose water

Put all the dry ingredients together into a muslin bag and add to the bathwater with the rose water.

milk bath

The classic: just add a few handfuls of powdered milk to the warm water and bathe like Cleopatra.

breast oil

Use this massage blend to tone and firm the breasts: the mustard oil makes the skin softer, while the powdered pomegranate rind has a firming effect.

ingredients
- 4 parts mustard oil
- 1 part dried pomegranate rind

Grind the pomegranate rind to a powder. Warm the mustard oil in a bowl over a pan of hot water. Mix the ingredients and leave to cool. Use the blend to massage the breasts with upward, circular motions, working outward from the nipples. Leave the oil on for at least 20 minutes, then rinse off with warm water and finish by splashing your breasts with cold water.

nail care

Whenever you're using oil, take a moment to rub some of it into your nails. Vata types often have pale, irregular nails that break easily. Pitta is linked with pink, oval nails that may be quite soft. Kapha nails are square and strong. All types can benefit from a hand cream of almond oil and honey.

hair removal

Women across Asia remove unwanted hair using the technique called threading. They hold one end of a cotton thread between their teeth, making a loop to lasso each hair, and tweak it out. This can be done professionally by beauty therapists. Easier to learn, and suitable for larger areas, is sugaring, using a mixture that is traditionally made at home. This can be made in large batches and kept in a jar. Sit the jar in hot water to soften it before use. It should last for a few months, as lemon is a natural preservative. You'll also need some strips of thick cotton, about 5–7.5 cm/2–3 in wide and 25 cm/10 in long.

ingredients
- 50 g/2 oz/4 tbsp sugar
- 30 ml/2 tbsp lemon juice

Simmer the lemon and sugar very slowly over a very low heat for a few minutes, stirring constantly, until they form a honey-coloured substance like sticky toffee. Experiment to get the consistency right: if it is too thin, add less lemon juice next time.

Allow to cool a little, then patch test to see if the temperature is tolerable. While still warm, spread on to the skin using a spatula. Place a cotton strip on the sugared area, press it down so that the warmth of your hands helps it to stick, and then pull off. On soft areas such as the calf, hold the muscle taut to prevent bruising.

▽ Practice makes perfect with sugaring, but the reward for your patience is silky smooth skin.

Shimmering tresses

◁ **The fragrance of jasmine and its delicate, waxy flowers complement the gleam of sleek, shining hair.**

△ **Neem has many healing properties, and is available in the form of powder, oil or leaves. It has long been used to improve hair condition.**

Historically, perhaps no part of a woman's body has aroused more adulation than her hair. Throughout the ages flowing tresses have been praised in poetry and celebrated in art. In some cultures hair is still hidden to avoid tempting men or angels. The fifth-century Sanskrit poet Bhartrhari described a woman's hair as a forest, enticing the explorer into unknown territory where love waits like a bandit to ambush him.

Indian women have always been proud of their shining hair. The ancient carvings of Mohenjo-Daro and Harappa show women with their hair magnificently styled and jewelled. Traders carried perfumes from one continent to another for noblewomen to scent their tresses, jewellers created gold clips to hold their hair in place, and village carvers made combs of wood or bone for themselves and their daughters.

Lustrous hair is one beauty available to most women. The rich anointed their heads with priceless unguents and twined strings of gems through their artfully arranged curls. But any woman can scent and enhance her hair with a simple flower-sprig.

hair treatments

Traditionally, people massaged their hair with oil to keep it healthy and counteract the drying effects of heat. Fragments of a dried tree resin called sambraani would be burned and the hair allowed to dry in its fragrant smoke after washing. Harsh shampoos and chemical treatments were unknown. Despite the range of hair products now available, many people are turning back to tried and tested formulas, some of which blend traditional knowledge with modern convenience. Instead of crushing leaves from the neem tree to enhance hair condition, for example, you can now pick up a bottle of neem shampoo or conditioner.

Hair and scalp problems may suggest a dosha imbalance, though they may also be

▽ **Use your fingers to comb the mixture through your hair down to the tips before rinsing out.**

aggravated by stress, harsh shampoos, excessive heating or air conditioning. Dandruff, with a dry and flaky scalp, is frequently caused by the drying effects of aggravated vata dosha. But if the hair is dull and the scalp red and inflamed, the imbalance is more likely to be pitta – which is the commonest cause of hair problems. An Ayurvedic practitioner may suggest herbal remedies and massage with particular oils to calm the aggravated dosha. Changes to the diet are likely to include more green leafy vegetables, salads, milk, fruits and sprouts, buttermilk, yeast, wheat germ, soy beans, whole grains and nuts.

blends to combat dandruff

These blends can be made in a screwtop glass jar and shaken to mix before using. The mixture should be worked into the scalp and left on overnight if possible; if not, wait at least 3 hours before washing your hair.

• 5 ml/1 tsp camphor added to 120 ml/ 4 fl oz/½ cup neem oil.

• 5 ml/1 tsp each castor oil, mustard oil and coconut oil.

• 1 part fresh lemon juice added to 2 parts coconut oil.

△ **Lime juice helps to soothe an irritated scalp and leaves hair with a lustrous shine.**

blends to soothe an itchy scalp

• 5 ml/1 tsp camphor added to 120 ml/ 4 fl oz/$^1/_2$ cup coconut oil. Massage the mixture into the scalp. Leave for at least three hours before washing off.

• Dried jasmine root, ground into a bowl of lime juice. Wash the hair and scalp with this mixture and rinse with lukewarm water.

rinses to add shine to the hair

• Squeeze a little lemon juice into a bowl of warm water and use as a final rinse.

• Add a little lime juice to a cup of rose water, add a cup or two of warm water and use as a final rinse.

egg conditioner

For dry hair, massage a beaten egg into the hair after washing and rinsing. Rinse out thoroughly.

rinse to prevent hair loss

Boil some neem leaves in water and leave to cool before straining off.

hot-weather conditioner

ingredients

• 1 egg

• 30 ml/2 tbsp castor oil

• 5 ml/1 tsp cider vinegar or wine vinegar

• 5 ml/1 tsp glycerine

To bring limp hair to life, mix the ingredients and beat well. Massage into the hair, leave as long as you like and wash out.

WHAT IS YOUR HAIR TYPE?

Like the rest of our bodies, our hair can show signs of our predominant doshas. If you're a dual-dosha person, you may feel that your hair seems to be out of line with your personality. How can a calm kapha have such dry, brittle hair? The answer is that your hair is reflecting your vata side while your inner self reflects kapha.

• If your constitution is mainly vata, you're likely to have dark, dry, coarse or frizzy hair that's prone to tangling, split ends and dandruff.

• Pittas are often blondes or redheads. They have enviable hair – fine and silky – but it needs looking after to prevent a tendency to go thin and grey before its time. It tends to be oily, but harsh shampoos make matters worse and can accelerate aging.

• People of kapha constitution may complain about their oiliness, but they have the least to worry about with hair that's naturally thick, glossy and wavy.

△ **Pitta hair rewards gentle treatment with silky sleekness. Don't be tempted to use harsh products that may cause thinning.**

△ **Kapha's fabulous mane grows long and thick at any age. If it shakes off efforts to control it, just revel in its exuberance.**

▷ **The traditional oil-based hair treatments used in India are particularly valuable for vata's dry hair, which is prone to tangling and splitting.**

Enriching oil treatments

Traditionally, Indian women regularly treat their hair with oil, using vigorous circular motions of the palms and fingertips to work it well into the scalp and down the length of the hair. They leave the oil in until they next wash their hair and then oil the hair again as soon as it dries. It's an intense massage treatment that stimulates the scalp as well as coating the hair shaft.

The lustrous, gleaming effect used to be admired in Western countries too. These days, we tend to prefer a just-washed look, replacing the hair's natural oils with conditioner. But for a change, why not try a pre-wash oil massage instead? After the massage, wrap a towel round your head, and leave it on for a few hours or overnight. You may need to vary the amount of shampoo you use. Why not also try leaving off conditioner for a while, to see whether you really need it?

warming and cooling oils

Oil is used to strengthen and nourish all kinds of hair, but like most Ayurvedic treatments it should be tailored to suit the person. Your choice should also be influenced by external conditions such as the weather or the time of year. Coconut oil is popular for head massage, as it is renowned for its nourishing and strengthening powers. But it also has a cooling effect, which means it's best used in hot weather. The same goes for oil infused with brahmi – a valuable herb that's believed to stimulate the brain as well as the body.

In the winter, use a warming oil such as mustard or olive. Mustard is very nourishing and has a strong heating effect, though it smells rather strong. Almond is more neutral but has a slightly warming effect.

Choosing the right oil for the time of year is part of the Ayurvedic rhythm. But if you're feeling out of sorts, your need to balance your dosha by using particular oils may override this consideration. If you use a cooling oil in winter, stay in a warm room and don't go out till you've showered the oil off and dried your hair. If you use a warming oil in hot weather, rest until you feel more comfortable with the temperature.

hair oil and your dosha

Vata's typically dry hair will revel in the luxury of black sesame oil, showing its benefits in a rich lustre. Pitta needs very gentle massage with brahmi oil or coconut oil, to stimulate the scalp without damaging the follicles. These two oils are good for all hair types.

If you're kapha, good hair is your birthright and the only thing that's likely to go wrong is an excess of oil – possibly because you scrub your scalp too vigorously or use harsh shampoos. Use sesame or mustard oil, but leave it on for only 30–60 minutes before showering it off. Avoid stimulating the scalp with intense massage or when washing your hair.

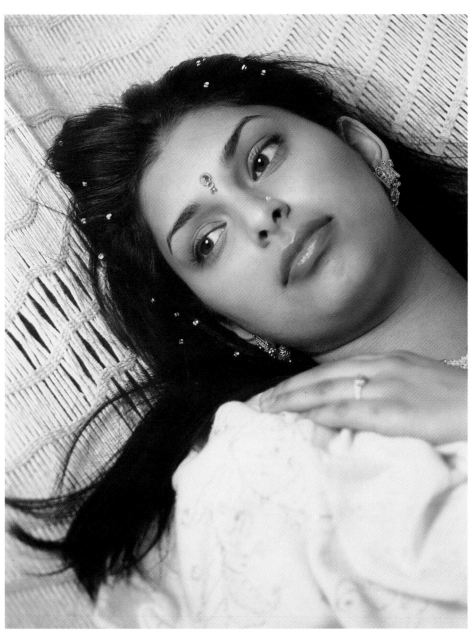

◁ **Luxuriant hair seems to come naturally to Indian women, whatever their dosha. Use of oil is one of their most effective beauty secrets.**

◁ If you don't want to leave oil on your hair for long, wrap your head in a warm, damp towel after applying it, in order to aid penetration.

▽ Gentle treatment brings out the best in fine flyway hair, so nurture it with the softest oil massage to help bring it back into balance.

warmth and penetration

Warming the oil before you use it on your hair can help it penetrate the hair shaft more effectively. Heat it very slightly in a non-metallic bowl over a pan of water. It should be no more than comfortably warm. Alternatively, wring out a towel in hot water and wrap it around your head – again ensuring that the heat is not uncomfortable – when you have applied the oil and again after massaging it in.

If you use a sauna or steam room, oil your hair before you go in and wrap it in a towel. This not only gives the oil a chance to penetrate more deeply, but it also protects the hair from the long-term drying effects of steam and heat.

hair and head massage

Why not combine an oil treatment for the scalp with a head massage, which Ayurveda recommends as part of your regular self-care routine? The series of movements aims to stimulate the body's systems, including glands, nerves and circulation, with anti-aging effects.

hair strengthening

If your hair is thinning or breaks easily, massage it with a strengthening herb-infused oil. This treatment is particularly recommended during pregnancy, to avoid the hair loss that plagues many women after childbirth.

ingredients

• 120 ml/4 fl oz/¹/₂ cup castor oil
• 550 ml/18 fl oz/2¹/₂ cups sesame or coconut oil
• 120 ml/4 fl oz/¹/₂ cup brahmi
• 120 ml/4 fl oz/¹/₂ cup amla
• 750 ml–1 litre/1¹/₄–1³/₄ pints/3–4 cups water

Mix the castor oil with the sesame oil (for vata-type hair) or coconut oil (for pitta) and add the brahmi and amla. Stir with a wooden spoon until the herbs have blended into the oil (you can warm the oil a little to expedite the process). Leave overnight, then pour the herb-infused oil, with the water, into an enamelled or non-metallic pan. Bring to the boil and simmer until all the water has evaporated. Remove from the heat and allow to cool, then strain through muslin or cheesecloth.

Supple
Sensuality

Indian women move with a natural grace

that makes them look like dancers. From

the steady tread of a country woman

carrying a basket home from market on

her head, to the curving hand and head

movements of a classical dance artist, every

movement reflects inner harmony. This

gracefulness can be within everyone's reach.

India's own form of exercise can shape your body,

clarify your skin and endow you with perfect poise.

Natural grace through yoga

As young children we all moved with unselfconscious grace, but from hunching over a school desk to slumping in front of a computer or television, many of us spend much of our lives with rounded shoulders and crumpled spines, and the heavy bags we carry often twist us to one side, too.

Most forms of exercise will help us look and feel better, but poor posture can sabotage a fitness regime, making exercise harder and leaving well-toned muscles further out of alignment than before. There is no such danger with yoga, and it is excellent for strengthening muscles and improving flexibility. In addition, its emphasis on lengthening and straightening the spine makes for perfect posture, creating an appearance of height and slenderness. Its regulated pattern of breathing lowers stress levels and eases tension from our faces as well as our bodies.

Yoga has become so popular in the West during the past few decades that we don't always remember where it came from. We

△ **Lengthening the spine and opening the chest is necessary if we are to help our cramped bodies regain a feeling of life.**

usually regard it as a set of flexibility exercises, or add it to a standard fitness regime as a stretch component. True, it is one of the best ways to build suppleness and delay the onset of old age. But yoga is far more than that, and in India it has always been closely linked with Ayurvedic medicine. Its name is Sanskrit for "union" or "connection": linking body, mind and the other non-physical levels to the universal mind. It has several elements, but the exercises generally practised in the West are what's called *hatha*, or physical, yoga.

Awareness of breathing is a central part of hatha yoga, and breath is synchronized with movement. Despite the effort you're putting in, this leads to a very calming, almost meditative rhythm that helps you push on through difficult parts. Pranayama – breathing exercises – form part of a standard yoga practice.

▽ **Working with a partner can help you keep your balance and move more confidently.**

SAFE MOVES

Hatha yoga was originally practised as an aid to meditation through controlling the body. Some movements, such as headstands, straight-legged body bends and backwards head rolls, can be dangerous for beginners. Others, such as stretches and twists, should not be forced. It's safest to learn from a qualified yoga teacher who has trained with one of the major organizations.

If you have health problems, don't take up any form of exercise before checking both with your own doctor and with an exercise expert who knows about medical contraindications. Yoga can bring great benefits to people with heart disease, back problems or arthritis, but they should take it up under the guidance of an instructor trained to work with these conditions.

◁ **A good teacher will ask about any injuries or health problems, ensure you are holding the poses correctly and also help you come out of them safely.**

styles of hatha yoga

Yoga's dynamic strength allows it to adapt while retaining its essential meaning. In recent years it has changed from a faintly exotic pastime to an everyday event. It is offered in many new forms, some of which are rediscoveries of ancient techniques.

Ashtanga is a vigorous form that builds up intense heat, intended to purify the muscles and organs, expel impurities and release hormones to nourish the skin. The fast sequences originally kept warriors fit, and they're an all-round exercise for flexibility, strength and cardiovascular fitness. It is aimed at people who are already very fit.

Bikram yoga quickly attracted dancers and celebrities to its creator's Beverly Hills studio. The idea is that practising a stripped-down core of movements in a room heated to above body temperature allows the muscles to stretch more, while impurities are washed out on a tide of perspiration.

Contact yoga is practised with a partner, requiring good co-operation and balance. Advanced practitioners may be able to do a headstand on their partner's head, but most stick to supporting each other's back bends or aiding a little more stretch.

Dru yoga is a very gentle, peaceful form that includes relaxation and working as a group.

Iyengar yoga is the best known form outside India. Detailed poses, or *asanas*, are

▽ **Your teacher can help you to increase your stretch while staying within safe limits.**

carried out with great attention to technique. It can feel strenuous, but it is done in a slow, controlled manner that should allow you to stop if you feel you're pushing your muscles too far.

Jivamukti is fast-paced and rigorous, but also includes chanting and meditation to help maintain the balance between physical and spiritual.

Kundalini yoga is an esoteric form that aims for enlightenment through the release of energy up the spine. This is achieved through stretching, breathing exercises, chanting and meditation.

Sivananda yoga, one of the least strenuous forms, considers the physical exercises to be part of a holistic lifestyle. It includes meditation and promotes a feeling of peace.

Vini yoga emphasizes safe movements and individual tuition, letting you adapt poses to meet your ability rather than trying to force yourself into them.

Yoga Vanda Scaravelli is a gentle adaptation of Iyengar, focusing on the spine. It uses gravity and the breath to undo tension in the body and awaken the spine.

▽ **Keep the neck long as you look up, visualizing space between the vertebrae. Letting your head slump back could harm your spine.**

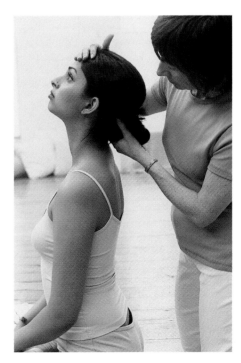

Find your fitness style

You don't need to read again that exercise is a vital component in any beauty regime. You may even be flipping guiltily past these pages, because you've come to see yourself as a hopeless fitness dropout. The Pilates class your friends rave about leaves you cold, and the last time you lifted a weight you felt like dropping it on the floor and running out of the gym. But don't despair: you could simply be following the wrong path for your dosha.

We all need to improve our cardiovascular fitness, increase flexibility, and build strength through weight-bearing exercise. But finding the right balance, and the right form of exercise, could be as simple as finding your true style. Even if you're perfectly content with your fitness routine – or lack of it – it's still worth considering whether you could make changes. When our energies are out of balance, we tend to slip further into the things that are causing the imbalance.

achieving balance

An energetic vata person may love running – an excellent and invigorating form of exercise. But when vata energy starts racing out of control, it's time to take another direction. Instead of arousing it further, turn to something slower and steadier, that will bring you safely back to earth.

A competitive pitta sportswoman may be way ahead of the field, but strangely unsatisfied by her achievement. Working up a daily sweat is just pouring fuel on her fiery nature. And it can be hard to persuade a relaxed kapha that exercise is a good thing when she feels fine without it.

It would be crazy to give up a form of exercise that you enjoy – it's hard enough for most of us to stick to a fitness programme. But Ayurveda suggests bringing more balance into your life, especially when your usual behaviour and routines are exacerbating any imbalances.

Sometimes our bodies instinctively know what's right for us at that moment, but sometimes we become set in ways that aren't the best. As you learn to know yourself better, you start to recognize the difference.

vata

You probably love lively exercise like dancing and running, but a typically speedy vata lifestyle can leave you feeling ungrounded. You also need to protect your joints from injury and build strength. As the most active of people, you're the least likely to need to join an aerobics class.

Bring your energies into balance with a steady, strengthening yoga style such as Vini. Iyengar is another good choice, so long as you're careful to recognize your current limits and don't risk harming vulnerable joints by excessive twisting or staying too long in a difficult weight-bearing pose. Instead of trying to force a stretch, let your muscles relax as you sink into a feeling of unhurried calm.

Walking, t'ai chi and Pilates are other useful exercises for you. Add some form of weight-training: the repetitive movements will leave your ever-active mind free to work out a new theory while you tone your abdominals. If these options sound slow and boring, give them a chance. As you become accustomed to this challenge you should start noticing a new smoothness in your movement as well as in your muscles.

▽ **Muscle-toning exercises such as Pilates are useful for vatas, whose high-speed metabolism makes aerobic exercise less of a necessity.**

pitta

Your competitive instincts lead you towards races and sports, but you need to avoid overheating, whether from exertion, a hot room or the midday sun. You could benefit from all yoga styles that increase flexibility without making you sweat. Concentrate on lengthening your muscles or easing gently into a deeper stretch without force or jerky movements, as in the yoga of Vanda Scaravelli. Working with a partner could help develop your co-operative instincts. The gentle routines of Dru or Sivananda yoga will promote feelings of peace that you may not have known for some time.

Swimming is ideal for your hot-blooded nature: the water helps balance your energies while you focus on your own steady progress. Cold-climate holidays give you a chance to enjoy skiing or snowboarding. Day to day, you need a moderate amount of exercise, with long walks providing an easy option.

kapha

You're naturally strong and healthy, and don't particularly like exercise, but you still need to build up flexibility and cardiovascular fitness. Though you reap the psychological benefits of taking life at a calm, steady pace, you need to build some energetic exercise into your routine.

With yoga, you're most likely to be motivated by a high-speed form that's fun and gets your body pumping out endorphins. Try Ashtanga or Jivamukti, which will also counteract your tendency to gain weight.

Any high-energy exercise class will give you the lively workout you need. Your strength makes you an asset in team sports, or you could take a salsa course.

△ Swimming is the perfect exercise for pittas: it's a rhythmic, calming motion that lets them work off plenty of energy without overheating.

▽ Anyone with kapha tendencies can have fun getting their exercise, and their stamina keeps them on the dance floor when others flag.

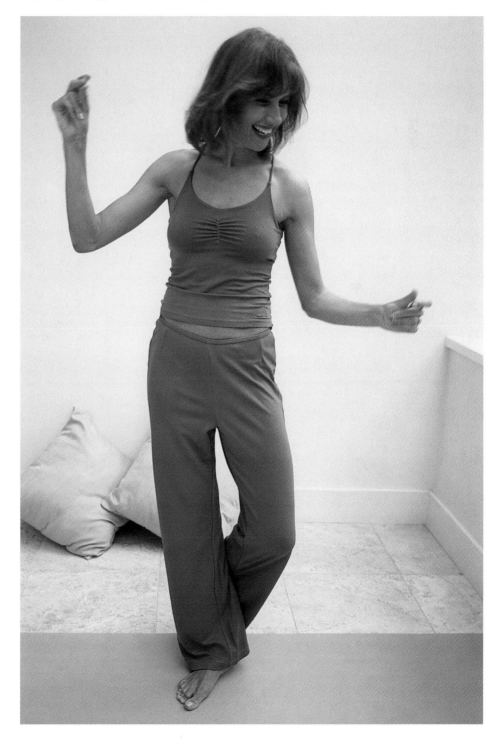

Move like a dancer

For most of us, brief bouts of exercise are interspersed with long hours of sedentary work, slumped in a chair and barely turning our heads. The effects show in our skin, our tired eyes and even our speech, from throats too constricted to allow our voices to be full and resonant.

All forms of yoga increase suppleness, allowing us to move more freely with a natural sensuality. Once we start practising yoga, the effects spread far beyond the hour spent twisting and stretching in the class. Straightening and lengthening the spine becomes a beneficial habit, changing the way we sit, stand, walk and talk. We hold our head level, as if suspended from the ceiling by a string, and the chin neither sags nor juts.

The asanas described on these pages are suitable for all doshas and are especially valuable for improving posture. In all cases you're aiming to lengthen and straighten your spine and limbs to rediscover a naturally upright stance.

the Mountain (Tadasana)

◁ **1** Stand with feet parallel and a little apart, arms by your sides. Lift and spread your toes, then plant them firmly on the floor. Keep your legs strong by feeling the front thigh muscles pulling up towards your groin. Tuck in your tailbone so that the front of your pelvis feels slightly higher than the back.

2 Lengthen your spine upwards while letting your shoulders and arms relax backwards and down. Imagine your head supported by a string from the centre of your scalp; your chin is level, leaving your throat comfortably open without compressing the back of your neck. Let your face relax.

3 Open your chest, without forcing your shoulders rigidly back. Let your stomach gently swell as breath fills your lungs, then tighten the abdominal muscles and expel all the stale air.

Standing Side Stretch (Ardha Chandrasana)

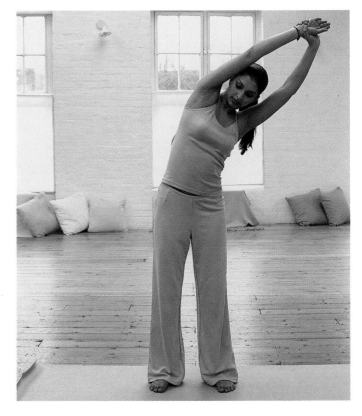

◁ **1** Starting in Mountain pose, take your feet a little further apart and slowly raise your arms above your head as you breathe in. Grasp your right wrist with your left hand as you breathe out.

▷ **2** On the next inbreath, lean to the left, facing forwards and bending sideways from the waist. Don't let your head, arms or torso flop; hold the position strongly and feel strength radiating from your fingers. Return to the centre on an outbreath and repeat on the other side, holding your left wrist.

the Tree (Vrksasana)

△ **1** Standing straight and looking straight ahead, take a moment to feel balanced and firmly rooted. Bending your right leg, place your foot as close to the top of your inside left thigh as you can comfortably reach, lifting it into position with your right hand if you wish. Stretch your right knee out to the side.

△ **2** To help keep your balance, fix your gaze on something motionless at about eye level. Spread out the toes of your left foot to grip the floor firmly. Breathing in, put your palms together with fingers pointing upwards as if making the Indian greeting *Namaste*. Try to hold this position for about 5 seconds, breathing naturally.

△ **3** On an inbreath stretch your arms straight above your head and turn your palms inwards. Feel the stretch from your raised hands to your feet, and the energy travelling the length of your body. Aim to hold for up to 20 seconds, breathing naturally. On an outbreath, bring your hands down, first to Namaste level, then down by your sides. Return your right foot to the floor and stand for a moment feeling grounded. Then repeat the exercise on the other side.

the Cow (Gomukhasana)

△ **1** Tuck your left heel beside your right buttock, trying to keep the knee on the floor. Cross the right knee over that leg and bring the right foot round beside you. If you find this difficult, sit with legs crossed and concentrate on the arm movements.

△ **2** Relax your right arm by your side then, on an inbreath, bring the right hand up between your shoulderblades. On the next inbreath, raise the left arm as if reaching for the ceiling. On the outbreath, bring your left hand down and try to grasp the right hand. If (like most of us) you can't reach at first, hold each end of a scarf. Hold the posture for around 10 seconds, breathing naturally, then on an inbreath raise the left hand again and bring both hands down beside you as you breathe out. Uncross your legs and stretch them out. Repeat on the other side.

Beauty from within

Why does your skin glow so beautifully when you surface from a swimming pool or return from a brisk walk? Any exercise that stimulates the circulation brings fresh oxygenated blood to the face, instantly enlivening the complexion. The long-term effects of regular exercise are just as clear – keeping the complexion fresh and strengthening the muscles that support the skin. The high-energy forms of yoga give your complexion a healthy boost that lasts long after you've showered and cooled down, but yoga's range of asanas includes several that stimulate circulation to the head without working up a sweat. Hold each of the poses for around 30 seconds, or as long as feels comfortable, and come out of them by retracing the steps described.

Downward-facing Dog (Adho Mukha Shvanasana)

In this position you should feel a stretch in your back and the backs of your legs, but don't force it, and don't try it without an instructor if you have trouble with your knees or lower back. If you're not very fit you may feel dizzy when you put your head down, so adapt the pose until you feel comfortable. (If the dizziness persists whenever you try this kind of exercise, get your doctor to check your heart and blood pressure.)

◁ **2** As you breathe out, try to straighten your legs by lifting your hips up and back. Keep your shoulders relaxed and breathe naturally. Your head should remain in line with your spine, not flopping down or pushed back. If you can straighten your legs without forcing your knees uncomfortably, increase the stretch by lowering your heels towards the floor. On an outbreath, try to lengthen your spine by bringing your hips further up and back.

△ **1** Kneel on all fours, with hips directly above knees and shoulders above wrists. Take time to feel well grounded, with toes tucked in below heels and fingers spread out, firmly gripping the floor.

the Lion (Simhasana)

This is a wonderful way of exercising your face, improving both circulation and muscle support. It firms the muscles of the face and neck, keeping wrinkles at bay.

▷ Sit with your legs crossed or kneel in a comfortable upright position. Rest your hands on your knees. As you breathe out spread your fingers wide apart, open your eyes as wide as you can and look up towards the centre of your forehead. Stick your tongue out and down as far as possible. Breathe out hard, making a loud, forceful "hah" sound. As you breathe in, draw in your tongue and relax your eyes and hands.

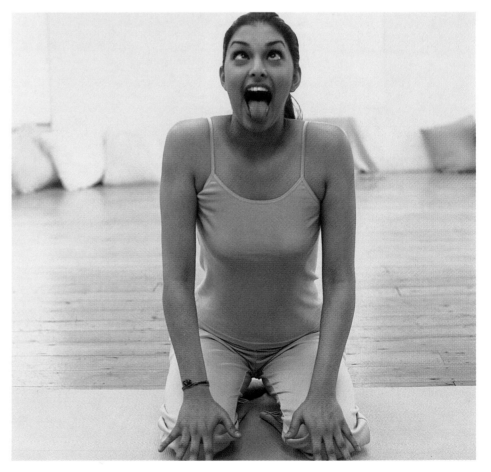

Standing Forward Bend (Uttanasana)

This useful asana revitalizes the complexion, tones the leg muscles, calms nerves and reduces vata energy.

◁ **1** Stand in Mountain pose, then move your feet shoulder-width apart. Breathe in and raise both arms above your head with palms facing in, feeling the spine stretch upwards.

△ **2** Breathe out as you bring your torso and arms slowly forward in a straight line, hinging from the hips and (to keep your back flat) leading with the chest. Go down as far as you can without straining your back. Keep the movement controlled to avoid harming your back, and bend your knees if necessary. Stay down as long as you feel comfortable, up to 30 seconds, breathing naturally, then, on an inbreath, bend your knees and unroll your spine vertebra by vertebra to come slowly up.

the Child (Murha Janusasana)

As well as improving circulation to the face and head, this is a very relaxing pose that eases the spine, making it ideal to follow more strenuous asanas.

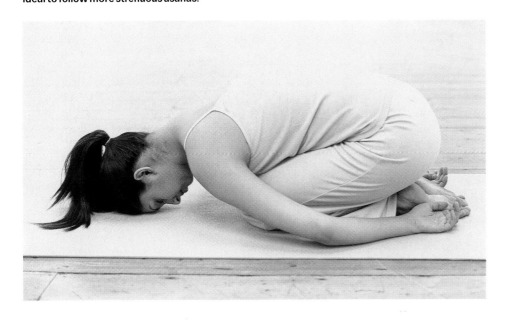

1 Kneel on the floor, sitting on your heels with legs together, arms relaxed by your sides and spine erect. As you breathe in, stretch your spine upwards as if pulled by a string from the top of your head and feel your chest and diaphragm expanding.

◁ **2** Breathing out, bring your body forwards face first, hinging from the hips without hunching the back. Bring your head down on to your knees or the floor in front. Rest your arms beside your body, palms up, on top of your feet if you can reach that far. Breathe naturally and feel your spine relax. This is a relaxation pose that you can hold for a couple of minutes, as long as you feel comfortable, before coming slowly up.

Body shaping

A sensuous shape relies on well-toned muscles. That means some kind of strength-building work, but many forms of strengthening exercise, such as weight-training, can create rather chunky muscles. Adding some stretch exercise is vital if you want to firm up without adding bulk, as fitness instructors always warn. The stretching element is built into yoga.

the Cat (Chakravakasana)

This tones muscles in the back, arms and buttocks and stretches the hamstrings.

◁ **1** Kneel on all fours with shoulders above wrists, hips above knees and soles facing upwards. As you breathe in, arch your back downwards so that your waist sinks lower than your hips and shoulders. Lift your head, without tipping it back – the length of your neck should be maintained.

△ **2** As you breathe out, come back to a central position. Continuing the outbreath, arch your back upwards and tuck your chin in towards your chest. Breathe in as you return to the central position and on to arch your back downwards. Repeat this movement slowly several times.

the Cobra (Bhujangasana)

This tones buttock muscles and pectorals. Don't risk damaging your neck by tipping your head too far back in this or any other backwards bend.

△ **1** Lie on your stomach with your head on one side resting on the floor, legs stretched out, with the soles of the feet pointing upwards, and arms by your side with palms upwards. Bend your arms and bring your hands beside your shoulders and, as you breathe in, slowly raise your chest. Keep your elbows beside your body, shoulders down and chest moving forwards. On an outbreath, push your palms down and raise your upper body as far as possible while keeping your pubic bone in contact with the floor. Look straight ahead, feeling the front of your body opening and expanding.

2 As you breathe in, raise your head slightly and direct your gaze upwards, but without tipping your head backwards. Relax the muscles in your back and buttocks, and feel your spine lengthen. Breathe naturally. Lower your gaze and look straight ahead again, then slowly lower your upper body to the starting position.

the Bridge (Setu Bandha)

In this asana, you're working on your hips and thighs.

△ **1** Lie on your back, arms by your sides with palms facing downwards. Bring your heels towards your torso, hip-width apart. As you breathe in, raise your buttocks as high as possible, pushing upwards with your pelvis till you are resting on your feet and shoulders. Tuck your chin in and let your head rest on the floor.

△ **2** If this is very easy, try an advanced version: with upper arms on the floor, bend your elbows and as you breathe out put your hands under your waist for support. Do not flop down on to your hands or push your spine up too high. If it's hard to keep your back raised, come down gently.

Lying-down Twist (Jathara Parivartanasana)

This works on trimming the waist while releasing tension from muscles in the back.

▷ **2** On an outbreath, lower your knees to the floor on one side and turn your head to the other. Hold for as long as is comfortable, then slowly come back to the centre on an outbreath, pause for a moment and repeat on the other side.

△ **1** Lie on the floor with arms outstretched, palms down. Bend your knees and raise them to your chest. Keep your neck and spine in a straight line.

the Warrior (Virabhadrasana) I, with arms raised

This pose tones the thighs, calves and chest.

1 Stand in Mountain pose, then move your feet sideways until they are about twice hip-width apart. Breathe in and turn your right foot through a quarter-circle to the right, placing your right heel in line with the left instep. Breathe out and rotate your body from the hips to face right.

▷ **2** Bend your right leg so that your knee forms a right angle, keeping the knee directly above the heel. Breathe in and raise your arms above your head until your hands are shoulder-width apart with palms facing in. Push your feet firmly into the floor and stretch up. Breathe out and lift your head slightly, without tipping it back, to look upwards. Breathe naturally and hold for a few seconds.

3 On an inbreath, lower your head again so that you are looking ahead. As you breathe out, bring your arms down by your sides, straighten your right leg and turn

your body to face the front again, with both feet pointing forwards. Keeping your legs wide apart, repeat the movements on the other side.

the Warrior II, with arms outstretched

△ Follow the instructions for Warrior I (left) for the leg movements for this version, but do not turn your body to the right or raise your arms above your head. Instead, trying to keep hips facing squarely forwards, stretch both arms out with palms facing down. Turn your head only, to look along your outstretched right arm.

Dynamic vitality

Different asanas can help you relax or feel more energetic, improve concentration or calm your mind. Calming poses include those where the body closes in on itself, such as the Forward Bends and the Child. For a surge of energy, you should work through dynamic positions such as the Lightning Bolt and the Warrior. Balancing asanas such as the Tree and the Eagle aid concentration and the Warrior poses promote inner strength. Any of the poses that release

tension, such as the Lying-down Twist or the Dog, can aid relaxation. But the classic relaxer is the Corpse.

The way you breathe is almost as important in yoga as the way you move. Keep your respiration steady and match your movements to the flow of breath, breathing in with an upward or outward movement, out as you go down or sink deeper into a stretch. You soon start to notice how it helps you keep a rhythm

to your movements. Aim to breathe out slightly more than you breathe in.

Breathing exercises, or pranayama ("controlling the life force"), form part of a yoga routine. In the Ayurvedic view, the breath carries the prana, or life force, around the body in thousands of channels; pranayama helps keep this flow steady and unobstructed. Because one of the main channels runs down the spine, good posture helps keep it clear.

Seated Forward Bend (Paschimottanasana)

▷ Sit upright on your tailbone with your legs together and straight out in front of you, toes up. On an outbreath, fold forwards from the hips to hold your ankles or your toes, without hunching your back. Ideally, keep your legs straight and bring your head down towards your knees, but let your knees bend if your back hurts, and don't force yourself to reach further than is comfortable. Hold for up to 30 seconds, then slowly return, on an inbreath, to an upright sitting position.

the Lightning Bolt (Utkatasana)

◁ **1** Start in Mountain pose, then breathe in as you raise your arms above your head. Breathe out and bend your knees. They should be no further forward than directly above your toes. Let your body slant naturally forwards, without rounding your back.

▷ **2** Be careful not to let your knees buckle inwards. Extend the arms in line with your torso. Breathe deeply three or four times, feeling the energy of the lightning bolt that your body forms from fingertips to toes. On an inbreath, return to Mountain pose.

the Eagle (Garudasana)

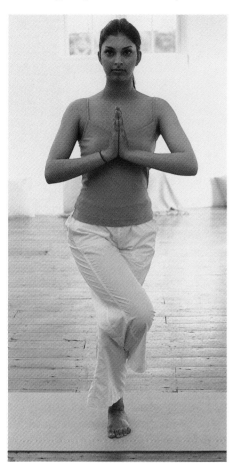

△ **1** Stand in Mountain pose and bring your hands into Namaste position. On an inbreath, bend your knees and wrap the right leg around the left, trying to hook your foot behind the ankle. To aid balance, focus your gaze on something still at eye level. Beginners can stay in Mountain pose and do the arm movements only.

△ **2** Keeping your shoulders relaxed, raise your arms in front of your shoulders on the next inbreath and cross the right elbow over the left. With thumbs at eye level, bring the palms together. Remain still, gazing at the thumbs and breathing normally. Be aware of the feeling of opening and stretching across your upper back; this is also excellent for relieving stiff shoulders.

the Corpse (Savasana)

△ Just as it sounds: lie on your back, arms by your sides with palms upwards and legs outstretched. Relax and let your feet roll outwards as your head seems to sink into the floor. If this makes your lower back ache, bend your knees upwards.

cleansing breath (kapalabhati)

This cleanses the entire respiratory system and freshens the skin. It also strengthens the muscles of the abdomen and aids digestion. It is considered so cleansing that its Sanskrit name means "making your skull shine". If you practise it every day your face should shine with health.

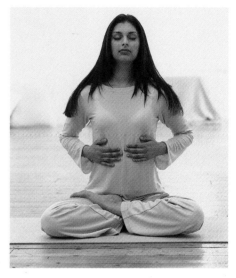

△ Sit with your back straight and breathe out hard in a series of short sharp exhalations through the nose. Tighten your stomach muscles as you breathe out, squeezing air out of your lungs. You won't need to make any effort to breathe in: when you relax the stomach muscles air will flow into the lungs naturally. After the tenth inbreath, breathe out for as long as you can and try to empty the lungs. Take a few normal breaths before doing another set.

bee breath (brahmari)

This is a relaxing technique that can send even insomniacs to sleep. It can also give you a deliciously sexy voice, releasing tension in the throat that causes harshness or squeakiness.

Sit upright, close your eyes and let a long outbreath lead naturally to a long inhalation. Breathing through your nose, make a continuous humming sound each time you breathe out. Relax and let it become a deep, rich sound. Focus your mind on this sound, which should continue the whole time you're breathing out.

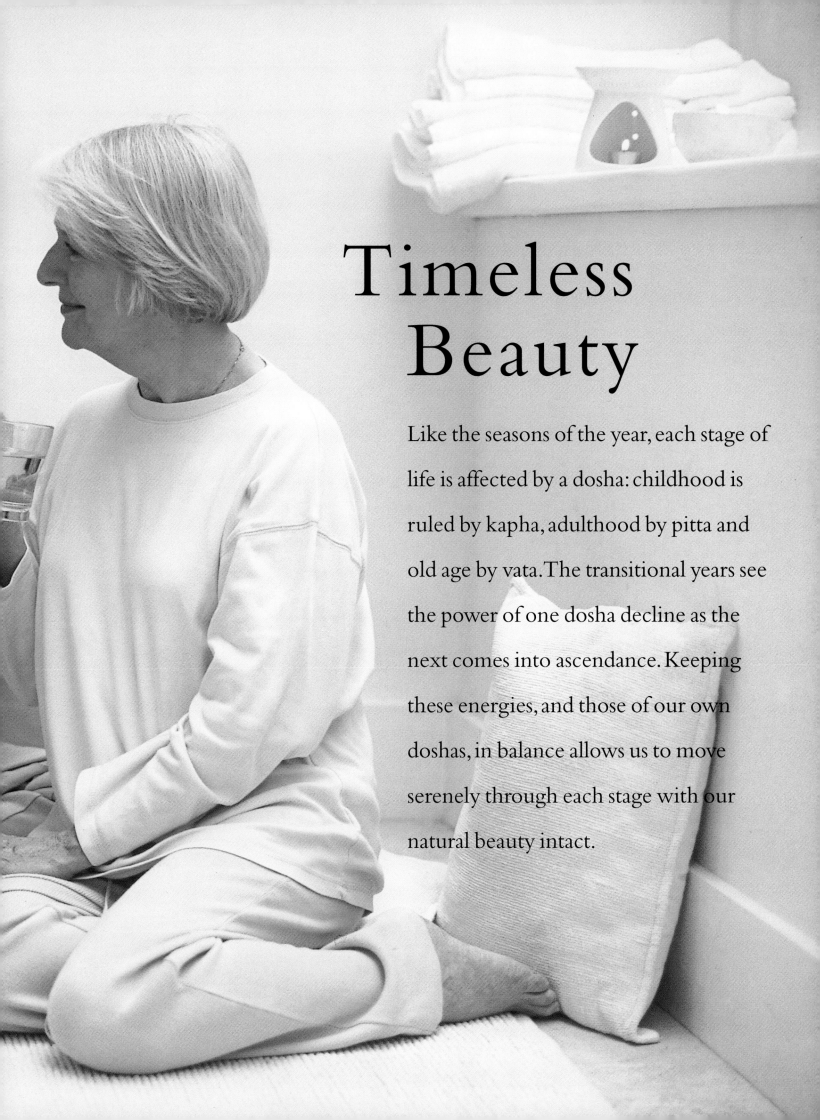

Timeless Beauty

Like the seasons of the year, each stage of life is affected by a dosha: childhood is ruled by kapha, adulthood by pitta and old age by vata. The transitional years see the power of one dosha decline as the next comes into ascendance. Keeping these energies, and those of our own doshas, in balance allows us to move serenely through each stage with our natural beauty intact.

The teenage transition

As children we had kapha's perfect skin, placid outlook and natural grace – not that we cared. Within a few years we're wondering what happened to those desirable attributes and wishing we could get them back. But by then we're already moving on into the pitta stage, which will last until the menopause.

Transitions are always a challenge, and – after birth – adolescence is the first big one. With depressive kapha and fiery pitta energies in conflict, our moods lurch from rage to despair. Since blood is a pitta element, the start of a period banishes premenstrual syndrome by reducing excessive pitta energy – but then hormonal changes make the skin erupt with acne and the hair turn lank. In Ayurvedic terms, the last burst of kapha energy turns skin into an oil well, ready to be ignited by pitta's fire. The body's toxic load of ama builds up too, and can find no way out except into the skin.

We slouch to disguise our embarrassing new height and breast shape (or lack of it), and loss of self-confidence can lead to problems such as eating disorders. Yet this is also a time of excitement and discoveries, as we move towards independence. Ayurveda's holistic teachings show us how to be our best now, and at every stage of life. The earlier we start, the more radiant health and confidence we gain to carry us through challenging stages.

Yoga routine

Carrying out this set of asanas every day should help clear your skin, keep your weight steady and give your body image a healthy boost. When you have time and energy, do all the positions instead of making choices. Keep your movements strong, feeling the energy coursing through your body and out to the tips of your fingers and toes.

 1 Start in Namaste then move into the Tree, to improve your balance – especially useful for days when you feel clumsy. Or move into the Eagle pose, to improve concentration and stretch the muscles of your back, counteracting the effects of working at a desk. Optional: return to the Mountain pose and do a Standing Side Stretch.

2 Try the Warrior pose, to shape legs and increase inner strength, helping you cope with mood swings and PMS, or the Lightning Bolt, for more energy.

3 Perform the Forward Bend, staying down for as long as you feel comfortable – up to 30 seconds – to stretch your hamstrings and bring fresh oxygenated blood to your face to clear skin blemishes.

4 Lie down and perform the Cobra.

5 Turn over and move into the Lying-down Twist, to tone your waist and let your hips swing as you walk.

6 Move into the Corpse. While you're relaxing after your workout, try to let your mind go blank and feel as if you're sinking into the floor.

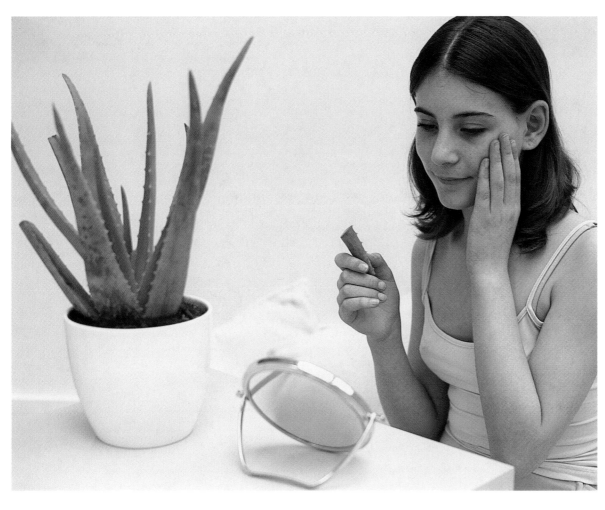

◁ Soothe spots and inflamed skin with the juicy pulp from an aloe vera leaf. It will leave your face feeling clean and supple.

feed your face

The skin blemishes that disfigure the teenage years are caused by an excess of kapha and, especially, pitta energies. Kapha increases oiliness, leading to blackheads, while pitta energy causes inflammation and eruptions. These can be counteracted by avoiding the rich, fried and highly spiced foods that aggravate pitta and – to a lesser extent – the sweet or salty foods that do the same to kapha. To reduce ama, eat food as fresh and unprocessed as possible. Junk food breaks most of the laws of Ayurveda and has cruel effects on teenage skin.

teenage skincare

When skin erupts, it's natural to feel desperate and scrub it with chemicals, but these often make matters worse. Instead, just keep skin normally clean and resist the urge to touch it. Dab spots with cream made from the antiseptic leaves of the neem tree – then leave them alone. For a very simple remedy, keep an aloe vera plant to break tips off, or buy the pure pulp. Fresh air is good for your skin, but don't sunbathe. Strong sunlight slows down oil production temporarily, but it may then go into overdrive to compensate. Skin cancer is a greater risk if you've been sunburnt in your teens.

SKINCARE RECIPES

Each of these soothing preparations for troubled skin should be spread over the face and left for 15–30 minutes while you relax. Rinse off thoroughly with warm water and splash with a gentle toner such as rose water.

FOR OILY SKIN:

• Beat an egg white until it is fluffy and add 5 ml/1 tsp tangerine juice.

• Mix 2.5 ml/1/2 tsp honey with 10 ml/2 tsp lemon juice. Mix to a paste with multani mitti (fuller's earth) and a little rose water. This should be removed after 15 minutes.

△ **Combat acne with plums mashed in almond oil.**

◁ **Fenugreek is used as a purifying herb – on the skin as well as in food.**

FOR ACNE:

• Boil 6 plums until soft, remove the skins and mash the pulp with 5 ml/1 tsp almond oil.

• Mix 5 ml/1 tsp each sandalwood powder and turmeric with enough milk to make a paste.

• Mix 5 ml/1 tsp either nutmeg or ground cumin seeds with water and spread on the affected areas only.

• Make a paste of fenugreek leaves and water, and spread on acne-prone areas. This can help prevent spots appearing.

Adult life: staying on top

Adulthood is pitta, ruled by the fiery dosha whose energetic influence sees us through our many tasks and responsibilities, not the least of which are the bearing and raising of children. At the busiest time of our lives, overwork can trigger a pitta imbalance, manifesting itself as irritability, impatience and heartburn.

dinacharya

Routines are a central part of Ayurveda, which teaches that living to a rhythm helps to keep us in tune with the energies inside and around us. Establishing an Ayurvedic routine, or *dinacharya*, is the first step to bringing the energies back into balance. It also makes it easier to sleep, exercise and eat healthily, helping to keep your weight steady and your skin clear.

• Wake up early – if not before sunrise, at least an hour before you have to leave home. Take a couple of minutes to visualize the day ahead and see it all going smoothly, then get up within about five minutes of waking.
• Give yourself a brief whole-body massage. If you use oil, leave it on for about 20 minutes before showering.
• Take 10–20 minutes to meditate and do some breathing exercises.
• Wash or shower, and splash your face and eyelids with cold water after cleansing.

△ **Daily cleansing is part of staying healthy, and gently scraping the tongue freshens your mouth.**

Clean your tongue with a special scraper, or use the edge of a teaspoon (kept for that purpose only).
• Drink a glass of water, cool or warm but not ice-cold, to aid digestion and help keep skin fresh.
• Do your yoga routine now if possible.
• Don't leave home without eating any breakfast. Clean your teeth and tongue after you have eaten, and try to do the same after every meal.
• Drink water throughout the day so you

never feel thirsty. However, it's best not to drink while you're eating.
• Have a good meal – preferably your main meal – at lunchtime. Eat mindfully, taking time to enjoy your food.
• Get some active exercise and some mental stimulation each day. If you work at a desk, go for a run or attend an exercise class. If you're running after children all day, read a book when you have a moment to yourself.
• If you didn't have time to do yoga in the morning, do it before dinner. Otherwise, meditate then.
• Eat a light evening meal, preferably early.
• Do 10–20 minutes' meditation if you didn't do this before eating.
• Go for a walk after you've eaten.
• Go to bed in time to allow yourself enough sleep. Most people need nine hours a night in their teens, decreasing to eight in their 20s, about seven in the 40s and an hour or so less in old age.

You'll be impressive if you stick to this routine every day – especially with children around. But using it as a basis helps you stay in control of your time and energy.

▷ **Balance your mental and physical routine. Read a book if you're always on your feet; go for a run if you do sedentary work.**

◁ **Don't stay in bed long after you've woken in the morning, but take a few moments to plan the day ahead and visualize it all going really well.**

▷ **Long before birth a baby is affected by your feelings. Gently massaging your abdomen nurtures the loving bond between you**.

pregnancy: glowing with new life

For someone used to being independent, pregnancy is a strange time as a new person's needs start encroaching on a woman's own. Some of the bizarre food cravings a pregnant woman experiences may be her body's attempt to balance her own doshas with the baby's.

The beauty benefits of pregnancy are a welcome side effect: glowing skin, voluptuous breasts and a mane of lustrous hair. Ayurveda can help you keep that glow. In India, a pregnant woman would be massaged by her husband and relatives. Gentle foot and ankle massage, with firm upward strokes, helps relieve swelling. After the fourth or fifth month, oil rubbed into the abdomen helps the skin maintain its elasticity, avoiding stretchmarks, and a backrub can wipe away tension from the face as well as the aching back.

Traditionally, pregnant women were encouraged to snack on sugared hibiscus flowers and rest as much as possible – with one exception: they swept the floors in a squatting position, strengthening the pelvic

area to prepare for childbirth. An antenatal yoga class will teach gentle exercises with the same aim.

Be cautious about massaging the back or abdomen during the early months, in case of miscarriage. Ayurveda recommends plain almond oil: if you want to use anything else, check beforehand with a reputable aromatherapist to find out which oils should be avoided during pregnancy.

If you're taking up yoga, make sure your class is run by a suitably qualified teacher. If you already practise yoga, take advice on how to modify your routine. Remember that not all pregnancies are standard, so seek medical advice if you have any concerns.

▽ **You and the baby need to rest. If you haven't got a large Indian family to cosset you, seize time for yourself and accept all the help you can get.**

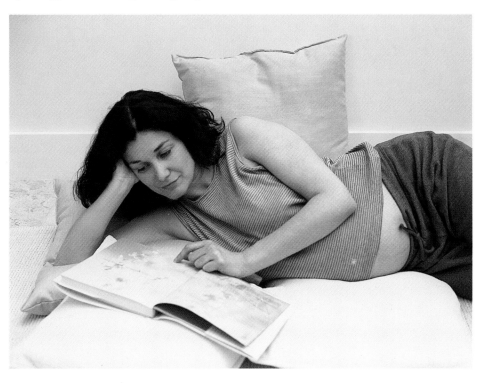

△ **Squatting can help to strengthen the pelvic floor, but in the later months of pregnancy it's safer to modify the pose, sitting on a low stool.**

yoga squatting pose

1 Stand with feet more than shoulder-width apart, toes turned out, and hold the hands in front of you in Namaste position.

2 On an outbreath, bend your knees and squat, keeping your spine erect. Try to put your heels on the ground if you can, but don't force this. Keep your knees as wide apart as possible.

3 If you've squatted low enough, bring your elbows down between your knees (fingers still pointing upwards), to encourage them further apart. Support your heels on books if they do not reach the floor, and your buttocks on a low stool or rolled towel if you're not comfortable squatting. Eventually you're aiming to put your heels on the floor.

TIPS

• Massage your hair throughout pregnancy and after the birth, to reduce the risk of hair loss caused by hormonal changes.
• Drink hot water with a slice of fresh ginger to relieve morning sickness.

The middle years

As pitta dosha starts to subside and vata increases, women reach the second great transition in life: the menopause. Though pitta is waning, it's no longer regularly reduced by the loss of blood during a period, so it may flare up in sweating and irritability. Heavy periods may be a sign that the body is trying to offload excess pitta. Toxic ama tends to build up as periods become irregular. This leads to lower back pain and an increased risk of growths on the reproductive organs.

Meditation helps combat the stress that magnifies some symptoms and triggers others, such as hot flushes. It's especially important to try to meditate in the morning, to leave the mind calm and able to organize the day's tasks.

Insomnia strikes many women as they reach the menopause. A regular bedtime routine helps to train the mind to turn off at the right time. Ayurveda also recommends going to bed during the kapha hours before 10pm. If this makes you wake up even

earlier, don't spend more than 10 minutes trying to return to sleep – get up and meditate instead.

Yoga practice is also important. Keeping a straight back and open chest allows you to breathe more fully, and weight-bearing exercise keeps bones strong. Add some form of exercise that leaves you slightly out of breath, such as brisk walking or low-impact aerobics. As well as keeping weight under control, this improves the skin.

changing tastes

Choosing the right foods is most important during the menopause, both to bring the doshas into balance and to meet the body's changing needs. Iron, for example, is no longer so necessary, whereas calcium is vital to keep bones strong.

Ayurveda's healthy living rules are made to meet beauty needs as well as promoting long life. The foods that keep the doshas in balance also promote clear skin and a slim, strong physique. Milk and cottage cheese, for example, pacify both vata and pitta while providing calcium and Vitamin D. Base your diet on fresh vegetables and fruit with some dairy foods, nuts, seeds and grains.

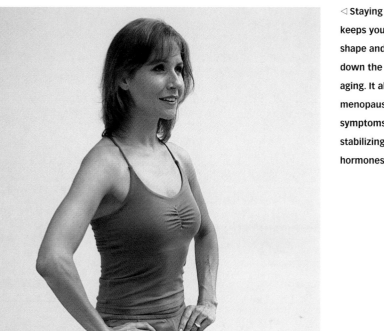

◁ Staying active keeps you in good shape and slows down the effects of aging. It also eases menopausal symptoms by stabilizing your hormones.

▷ Changes in your body's hormones can make this stage of your life difficult, but an Ayurvedic remedy will help to balance them.

△ Soothe vata with gentle oil massage, brief steaming and a cooling facepack.

save your skin

As vata dosha increases with age, its drying influence causes lines, wrinkles and thinning of the skin. Milk, honey and yogurt help to lubricate the skin from the inside, keeping it youthful.

Oiling the skin and then steaming reduces excess vata, making this a suitable beauty treatment throughout life. Because fine facial skin can be damaged by too-frequent steaming, it should be done only once or twice a month. Regular use of nourishing facepacks can help to keep the skin properly moisturized, slowing down the aging process.

seeing clearly

Delay the need for reading glasses with some eye exercises. (If you wear contact lenses, remove them first.) Sit with your spine straight and shoulders relaxed, and look straight ahead. Keep your head still while doing the exercises. Hold each eye position for 3–5 seconds and repeat three times.

△ **1** With your forefingers at eye-level in front of you, hold one at arm's length and the other half that distance away. Focus on one, then the other.

2 Look diagonally up to the right, then down to the left. Look diagonally up to the left, then down to the right. Look as far as you can up, down, left and right.

3 Rub your hands together to warm them, then cup your palms over your eyes for a few minutes.

mula bandha: yogic exercise for the pelvic floor

Many women approaching the menopause find their pelvic floor muscles have weakened, giving little or no warning of the need to urinate. Simple exercises can banish this embarrassing problem. Begin by tightening your anus, then add a squeeze in front as if stopping yourself urinating, and hold both squeezes while trying to lift the pelvic floor. It's a tiny movement. If you lay your forefinger flat along the perineum – the strip of skin between vagina and anus – you should feel a very small lift. Start by doing this three or four times after using the lavatory (don't try to stop the flow of urine as this can cause bladder problems), then practise it for 5 seconds at a time, for example while holding any yoga pose.

Moving forward

This is a time when many people – whose earlier lives may have been too hectic for regular practice – discover the benefits of yoga. Notice how much more confidence they have than most older people. This confidence is based on a strength and suppleness that makes them far less prone to accidents and falls.

From as early as the 30s, muscles start to stiffen and joints lose their range of movement. As the years pass, even people with good posture start to walk and turn less smoothly. Long-term yoga practice can delay the onset of these restrictions by many years, but taking up yoga in later life can also reverse some of the changes age has made.

By encouraging correct posture and maintaining flexibility in the spine, it helps to delay the effects of aging. Starting each day with a routine lasting 20–30 minutes leaves you in good shape and gives you time to clear your mind for the day.

▽ **Take care of your body, not by reducing activity but by ensuring that all the movements you make are beneficial. Squatting instead of bending, for example, reduces the risk of back pain at any age.**

TAKE IT EASY

If you have any medical conditions, check with your doctor before starting any kind of exercise and consider taking a remedial yoga class. In particular:

• Don't do inverted poses such as the Standing Forward Bend and the Downward-facing Dog if you have a blood pressure or heart condition. If you feel at all dizzy in any pose, come out of it gently and sit down.

• If you have arthritis or osteoporosis, beware of poses that put weight on your wrists, such as the Downward-facing Dog.

• Don't do the intense straight-legged bends and backward head-rolls that advanced yoga practitioners carry out. These can injure your spine. In any bend it's better to keep your knees soft, even slightly bent, and concentrate on gently rolling your spine down.

• After a yoga session you should be aware of the muscles you've worked, and may even feel a bit stiff over the next day or so when you're new to the practice. But your joints shouldn't hurt and any stiffness should wear off after a couple of days. If you do experience any pain, stop practising and see your doctor.

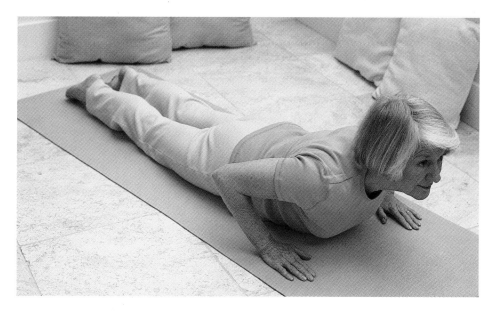

daily yoga routine

You should include asanas from each of the main groups, to work all parts of the body: standing, sitting and lying down; back bends, forward bends and twists. The following is a gentle and effective series suitable for older beginners.

1 Warm up by performing the Cat movement several times to get your spine working.

2 Stand up in the Mountain pose, to centre you and help keep your balance steady. As people age their sense of balance starts to fade, and it is this as much as loss of strength that leads to potentially dangerous falls. Keeping a good sense of balance gives you the same confident stride you had when you were young.

3 Move into the Standing Side Stretch. Check that you are breathing naturally and in rhythm with your movements: in as you lean downwards, out as you come up. Return to the Mountain pose and take a moment to feel centred again.

▽ **4** Now move into the Standing Forward Bend, keeping your knees slightly bent if you are new to this. If you feel any strain on your back, just move forwards enough to put your hands on a support such as a stable piece of furniture. Concentrate on keeping your back flat and your head in line with your spine.

△ **5** Return to the Mountain pose for a few moments, then lie down on your stomach and move into the Cobra pose. Keep your elbows bent and focus on opening your chest, letting your shoulders sink down and back, away from your ears. When you look upwards, do not to let your head tip back. You're aiming for a natural curve at the neck, without compressing the vertebrae. The same goes for the lower back, don't push yourself up with straight arms and an unnatural arch in your lumbar spine – it's the thoracic vertebrae in your upper spine that need to move.

6 Lower your chest and come smoothly out of the Cobra, then push your hips back and bend forwards into the Child pose, relaxing your spine by letting it curve in the other direction.

7 Move into a kneeling position and into the Dog pose.

8 Next, go into the Bridge, to increase flexibility in your spine. Keep your heels and your arms on the floor, with your palms facing down. You are aiming for a gentle curve in your spine.

9 Roll on to your side and sit up, then move into the Cow pose. This is meant to promote long life, because it opens your chest and stops your lower back stiffening. If you find the leg position difficult, simply sit or kneel with your spine straight.

10 Complete your routine by relaxing for a few minutes in the Corpse pose. Come up by rolling on to your side.

The Food of Life

A gift from heaven and earth, the food
we eat can nourish our spirits as well as
our bodies. Eating well enhances
beauty and preserves youthful vitality;
it's also a sign of healthy self-respect. In
Ayurveda, a meal prepared with love is
a blessing to those who cook and those
who eat.

Eating well

For many of us, food is at best simply fuel, at worst an enemy. Modern cook books set standards unknown to previous generations, yet most of the food we eat is commercially prepared. Nearly half of us are on a slimming diet at any given time, yet our average weight is rising steadily. No wonder so many of us view food with anxiety.

The Ayurvedic outlook is like a breath of sattvic fresh air. It teaches that eating is a pleasure, and one that does nothing but good. This approach doesn't lead to binge-eating; instead, it means putting a little time and thought into preparing food from fresh ingredients, then savouring it as you eat.

The freshness and quality of the food are important, since unwholesome ingredients create ama, or toxins, in the body. A diet that is based on meat, alcohol, processed foods, dairy products and white sugar and flour produces a lot of ama, leading to disease, bad breath, dull skin and unhealthy hair, while fresh, natural foods give you energy and vitality, and let your natural beauty shine through.

Ayurveda further emphasizes the need to digest food properly, since poor digestion leaves by-products that can also develop into ama. That's why each dosha type needs to eat a slightly different range of foods – those that they're most easily able to digest.

cooking with love

In today's speedy world we often feel too rushed to cook with fresh ingredients. But the steady rhythm of chopping vegetables and stirring pots can create a calm space in the day. And Ayurveda's simple recipes take little time to prepare.

In a traditional Indian household, the kitchen is an almost sacred place. Since everything in creation is deemed to have a soul, everything is entitled to be treated with respect – especially food, which imparts its life force, or prana, to the eater. Followers of Ayurveda believe that the feelings you experience as you cook enter the food and

△ To Ayurveda, almonds are full of prana; in Western terms they're rich in Vitamin E, calcium and beneficial fats – either way, a perfect snack.

affect anyone who eats it. So don't resent the time you spend cooking. If you enjoy creating a dish, feel nothing but love for those who are going to eat it (including yourself) and look forward to eating it, you'll be endowing the food with health benefits that can't be bought.

food basics

The mainstays of your diet should be fresh fruit and cooked vegetables, grains, nuts and seeds. Add salads and certain animal foods, depending on your dosha. Locally grown organic produce in season is the most natural, as long periods in transport or storage reduce nutritional value.

Meat and dairy produce should be organically produced. Factory-farmed animal foods are risky even by Western standards: they may be diseased or contain drug residues. But such foods are doubly harmful by Ayurvedic standards: the miserable lives of the animals produce low-quality prana, and your action in supporting intensive rearing creates bad karma.

Followers of Ayurveda are frequently vegetarian. Plant foods are full of prana and organic choices are best, as their chemical-free growth causes no harm either to them

or to the environment. These are the most physically and spiritually nourishing foods you can find.

how to eat

• Eat at regular times, leaving at least four hours between meals.

• Don't eat unless you're hungry. If you have no appetite, wait until your next meal time, drinking warm water in between. But don't go without food for more than a day.

• Always sit down to eat, and don't watch television, read or have emotional conversations during the meal.

• Eat slowly and savour food. This stops you over-eating, since it takes a while for your brain to register that you've eaten enough.

• Try doing a mindfulness meditation while eating. Focus your attention on the food: its colours, shapes, smell, texture and taste. You're less likely to overeat when your mind's on your meal.

• Eat raw fruit alone, not as part of a meal.

• Fast on fruit and vegetable juices and water for one day a month.

▷ Fresh organic fruit and vegetables are the mainstay of an Ayurvedic diet, good to eat without harming the earth they came from.

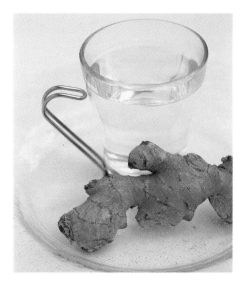

△ Ginger tea is renowned for strengthening the digestion and alleviating feelings of nausea.

what to drink

• Drink enough water to ensure that your urine is always a pale yellow colour: up to 2 litres/3¹/₂ pints a day is beneficial. Warm or hot water is best, and Ayurveda doesn't recommend drinking ice-cold water.

• Other healthy drinks are herbal teas, milk (depending on your dosha), fruit juices and vegetable juices.

• Ginger tea strengthens *agni*, the digestive fire. Warm water also aids digestion and should be drunk throughout the day.

• Choose healthy beverages more often than alcohol or stimulants like tea or coffee.

▽ Cranberry and apple juice are both full of vitamins. Dilute fruit juices with water for the best effects on the body.

The inner qualities of food

The gunas, or qualities, of foods are as important as their taste and nutritional value. All aspects of nature contain these inner properties – sattva, rajas and tamas – and therefore affect our own gunas whenever we come into contact with them. Since the food we eat becomes part of us, its guna has a particularly strong effect.

sattva

Few people attain the sattvic state of enlightenment, but when we approach it we're fully alert, clear-thinking and compassionate. Sattvic foods, the ones closest to that state themselves, help us towards it. They are the lightest and most wholesome ingredients, close to their

◁ **Light, healthy drinks and foods help you towards the sattvic state, in which you are peaceful and unburdened by negative feelings.**

natural state, such as fresh fruit and vegetables, honey, nuts and whole grains. The lighter dairy products – milk, yogurt and butter – are also sattvic. In keeping with Ayurveda's non-violent ethic, the most sattvic food causes no harm, so the best diet is based on organic fruit and vegetables, locally grown to reduce the environmental costs of transport, and organic dairy produce from animals kept in humane conditions.

rajas

The rajasic state is turbulent, always on the go and easily irritated. Rajasic food is the kind that fuels the go-getting Western world, and each time we eat it it adds to that tendency in us. Rajasic food is not bad, because we do need some stimulation, but since Ayurveda values peace more highly than profits, it recommends eating it in smaller quantities. Following that advice will do your body as much good as your soul, since rajasic food is the most likely to cause heartburn. If you have any tendency to be aggressive, cut down on it still further. It's high-protein, high-energy fuel. Rajasic

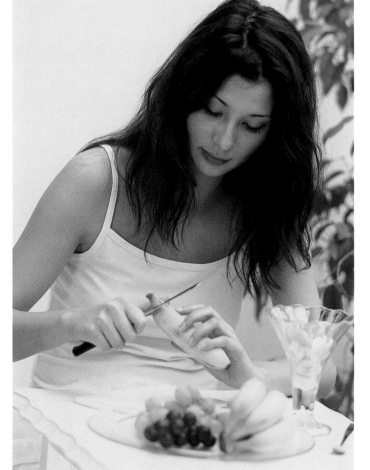

◁ **Fruit pacifies vata and pitta doshas and – especially when cooked – makes a healthy substitute for the cakes and sugary foods that can aggravate kapha.**

▷ **Rajasic foods fuel the Western lifestyle that leads to stress and burnout. Snacking adds to the ill effects, so take time to eat nourishing food.**

▷ We need high-protein foods to build our physical strength and give us rajasic energy. They only cause harm if, as in the average Western diet, we eat too much of them.

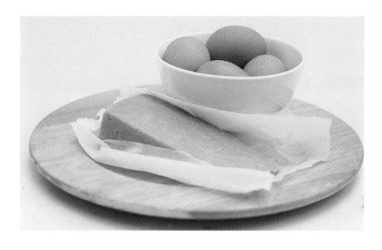

foods include meat, fish, eggs, hard cheese, hot peppers, sugary foods and root vegetables, along with anything that has been fried, pickled or highly spiced.

tamas

The tamasic state of mind is lethargic, ignorant, selfish and dull. It is fuelled by processed foods, artificial flavours or sweeteners, chemical preservatives, factory-farmed meat and dairy produce, and anything mass-produced without respect or made from low-quality ingredients. Meaty junk food is about as tamasic as food can be. Food that's stale and has lost its life force is tamasic too. For this reason, Ayurveda recommends cooking food fresh every day rather than using leftovers. Alcohol falls into the tamasic group, since although it's a stimulant at first it soon has a dulling effect.

▽ Mass-produced junk food has tamasic effects, but homemade cakes are a treat: moderation, quality and individual needs are important.

▽ Alcohol pushes us away from the sattvic state by causing confusion, damaging health and promoting aggression and laziness.

GHEE

Clarified butter, or ghee, is not only a mainstay of Indian cooking but an important Ayurvedic health product. You can make your own, though it may not taste quite the same as the product bought in Indian shops, which is often made with yogurt. If you have high cholesterol and don't normally eat animal fats, check with your doctor. If you can't use ghee, substitute vegetable oils.

To make ghee, put 1 kg/2¼ lb unsalted organic butter in a heavy pan and heat slowly, stirring constantly, until melted. Turn up the heat and let the butter froth for a few moments, then reduce the heat and

the six tastes

Ayurveda recognizes six flavours, which affect the balance of doshas. We all need all of them, but in differing amounts. You don't need to give up any of your favourite ingredients completely; if they're in a group that increases your dominant dosha, just eat less of them or prepare them in a way that makes them more suitable, such as tossing salad in a rich dressing to reduce its vata-raising properties.

• **Sweet:** increases kapha, reduces vata and pitta. Sweet-tasting foods such as honey, cucumber, dried fruit, most fresh fruits, and foods that become sweet when cooked, such as apples and onions. High-protein foods such as meat and nuts. Fats and oils. Butter, ghee and milk. Rice.

• **Sour:** increases kapha and pitta, reduces vata. Vinegar, pickles and aged food. Yogurt and cheese. Tomatoes. Citrus fruits.

• **Salty:** increases kapha and pitta, reduces vata. Salt, soy sauce.

• **Pungent (spicy):** increases vata and pitta, reduces kapha. Chillies, sweet peppers, many herbs and spices.

• **Bitter:** increases vata and reduces pitta and kapha. Most salad leaves and green leafy vegetables. Fenugreek and a few other bitter herbs. Coffee, chocolate.

• **Astringent:** increases vata and reduces pitta and kapha. Beans, peas, chickpeas, lentils. Cauliflower, broccoli, fennel, asparagus, chicory, aubergines (eggplant), celery, Savoy cabbage. Tea.

simmer gently, uncovered, for about 30 minutes, until transparent. Skim off the froth and any impurities and strain through muslin or cheesecloth, discarding the milky solids. Leave to cool and store in the refrigerator.

△ Golden richness with a sweet, nutty taste.

Diet and your dosha

Each dosha type is pacified or aggravated by different foods, so the food you eat can help to balance your constitution. Try to eat something from each of the six taste groups every day, with most of your intake coming from the groups that pacify your dosha.

the vata diet

Vata is pacified by sweet, sour and salty foods, but aggravated by pungent, bitter and astringent tastes. Raw food tends to increase vata. Try to balance your dry, cool, light constitution with foods that are hot, oily and heavy, such as soups and rich stews. Bananas, grapes and all sweet fruits are good, and meat suits your constitution better than most.

Natural foods are particularly important to vata, since it is aggravated by artificial additives. Most dairy foods suit you, but yogurt is best diluted: try mixing it with water, pure rose water and some honey or chopped fruit, or with water and a little salt to make the Indian drink called lassi.

Though many herbs and spices fall into the pungent category, they're only used in small amounts, so enjoy the warming qualities of spicy foods, though chillies are generally not recommended, since they're considered very dry.

▽ **If it's a hot day but you need to pacify vata, drink a refreshing glass of sweet or salty lassi.**

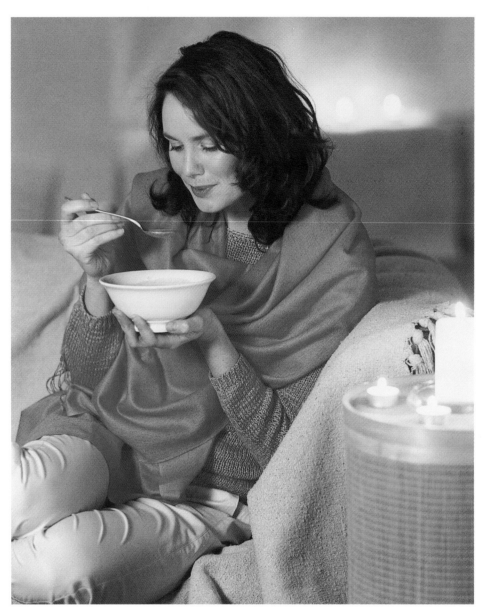

△ **Warmth and comfort soothe excess vata: a cosy room, a quiet evening, a bowl of rich soup.**

Toss salads in mayonnaise or rich dressings containing oil or coconut milk. You can use cooked ingredients to make a warm salad. If you like vegetables from the bitter and astringent taste-groups, cook them with oil or ghee. Ghee will also aid your digestion, which tends to be irregular. Anything light, dry and cool will increase vata, so you should avoid foods like crisps (potato chips), popcorn, dried fruits and undressed green salads.

Though sweet natural foods are good for vata, white sugar and white bread are too dry and light. Alcohol, tobacco and recreational drugs in general have strong vata-inflaming effects and should be avoided altogether or reduced to a minimum.

VATAS COULD TRY…

- Porridge with milk and honey.
- Roasted/stir-fried meat and vegetables.
- Stews cooked with ghee or oil.
- Cooked soft fruit with cream.

the pitta diet

The tastes that help to balance pitta are sweet, bitter and astringent. It is aggravated by those that are pungent, sour or salty. Pitta-pacifying foods are cold, heavy and dry.

Pitta dosha can make you digest your food too quickly, leading to poor absorption. Since Ayurveda teaches that good digestion is the foundation of good health, it is important to strengthen agni, the digestive fire that governs the metabolic processes. Some agni-strengthening foods tend to increase pitta too, but ghee is ideal: it balances pitta while increasing agni. To improve digestion, try to eat slowly in peaceful surroundings at regular times, without overeating. Don't have high-protein food late in the evening. Do take some time to relax after a meal.

Almost all vegetables are good for you, and most fruits that are not sour. Eat plenty of raw food and salad (other than tomatoes). The few vegetables that may not suit you include beetroot, carrots, aubergines (eggplant), garlic, onions and spinach. Chillies, salt and highly spiced food add too much fuel to pitta's fire. Instead, experiment with the cooling tastes of basil, coriander (cilantro), dill, fennel and turmeric, and other mild-tasting herbs. Eat only small amounts of concentrated protein such as red meat, seafood and eggs. Stimulants of all kinds aggravate pitta, so cut down on alcohol and coffee and avoid recreational drugs of any kind.

▽ **Excessive pitta heat is cooled by raw foods such as fruit, mild herbs, and vegetables such as broccoli.**

PITTAS COULD TRY...
- Cool stewed apple with pumpkin seeds.
- Green salad with fresh asparagus, drizzled with extra virgin olive oil.
- Rice and beans.
- Ice cream with fresh figs or blackberries.

△ **A salad is the ideal pitta lunch.**

the kapha diet

Kapha is balanced by pungent, bitter and astringent tastes, but aggravated by those that are sweet, sour or salty. Foods should be dry, light and hot.

The kapha constitution tends to be cold, so needs warming foods: freshly cooked, spicy or piquant with chillies. Include plenty of vegetables, cooked and eaten hot. Almost all vegetables are good for you, though sweet potatoes can be a little heavy and cucumber has a cooling effect.

You can improve your sometimes sluggish digestion by strengthening agni, the digestive fire. This can be achieved by eating

▽ **Gourmet kaphas can liven up their cooking with chillies, which provide an invigorating heat.**

cloves, pepper (black or cayenne), mustard, cinnamon and horseradish.

The cold nature of salads makes them less suitable for kapha, especially in winter. But don't rule them out completely: choose warm salads, or leaves with a sharp or mustardy taste, but don't smother them in dressing. You have a free hand with almost all herbs and spices, so use these flavourings instead of oils and fats.

Cut down on heavy foods such as wheat, red meat and cheese; lighter alternatives are barley, poultry and cottage cheese. You may have a taste for sweet or salty foods, but these should play only a minor role. Processed foods are high in fat or sugar, and "lite" versions just substitute artificial sweeteners. So leave them on the supermarket shelves and let your natural kapha cooking skills loose on the huge range of real foods.

KAPHAS COULD TRY...
- Cooked buckwheat with cranberries and sunflower seeds.
- Warm salad of raw baby spinach leaves and organic chicken.
- Spicy homemade curries rich with seasonings instead of oil.
- Pears stewed with ginger.

△ **Kaphas can enjoy almost all spices.**

Aging
Naturally

The fight against aging

The quest to extend the human life span is nothing new; scientists have long searched for ways to prevent aging and cure life-threatening illnesses such as cancer. Significant progress is being made in the field of gerontology and it is likely that in the future we will be able to slow the aging process down and live actively into old age. For example, in 1999, Italian researchers at the European Institute of Oncology in Milan published findings regarding the existence of a genetic defect in mice that causes them to live a third longer than other mice. The mice ate a normal diet and had a normal body weight but they lacked a gene for a specific protein. The implications of this finding for human life spans is the focus of intensive research.

taking care for your health

As you grow older it is important to be aware of the changes that take place in your body. You need to know how to prevent problems occurring and how to respond to them when they do. Taking responsibility for your own health and wellbeing gives you a powerful sense of control and self-confidence. However, this does not mean excluding healthcare professionals. For example, tell your doctor if you are taking herbal medicines. Other factors which may help include:

• Listening to your body and responding appropriately.
• Learning about complementary therapies and how they can help you prevent and treat health problems.
• Exercising regularly and concentrating on staying flexible and active rather than "going for the burn".
• Eating plenty of fruit and vegetables.
• Understanding the age-related changes that affect each body system. Learn which changes can be prevented, which ones should be accommodated and which changes may be early warning signs of health problems.

positive avoidance

Many of the harmful aspects of life have been identified, which means that we can now make a positive effort to avoid the things that cause us harm. For example, stress, cigarette smoking, drinking too much alcohol and long-term exposure to the sun and pollution are five of the major contributors to the aging process. Even if we eat healthy food, exercise regularly and have plenty of sleep, these factors will still have an adverse effect on the body.

Fortunately, it is comparatively easy to avoid cigarette smoking, excessive alcohol consumption and exposure to the sun. It is less easy to avoid pollution and stress; these are things that we need to tackle collectively, and this is now recognized and taken seriously by scientists, employers and governments. Also, even if can we cannot avoid stress and pollution there are ways of mitigating their effects on the body. There is a wide range of complementary therapies that can help us to relax and there is some evidence that taking antioxidant supplements can mitigate the damaging effects of environmental pollution.

complementary therapies

In the past, remedies for illness were passed down from one generation to the next in a strong tradition of herbal medicine. Although people may not have known how plant remedies worked, they remained tried and trusted ways of treating illness. For example, St John's wort was used as an antidepressant long before science taught us about serotonin, a brain chemical that affects mood. A report in the *British Medical Journal* stated that St John's wort has fewer side effects than imipramine, a widely prescribed antidepressant.

▽ **Acupressure can be particularly helpful for pain control, treatment of common ailments and boosting the immune system to help protect the body from disease.**

△ **St John's Wort is a natural antidepressant, but prolonged use may cause photosensitivity.**

Although conventional medicine remains the first option for many people during sickness, there is a move towards complementary therapies that treat the body as an interdependent whole rather than a collection of individual parts. It is now thought that many plant remedies are effective because they contain ingredients that work in concert with one another. In contrast, most Western drugs simply isolate the active ingredient in a plant.

Herbalism is just one of many types of complementary therapy available. Other types of recommended treatment include aromatherapy, massage, hypnotherapy, reflexology, dietary medicine and acupuncture. Complementary therapies are now recognized by many doctors and scientists as being valuable aids in assisting the body to fight illness and aging .

▷ **As we age our bodies become less supple and taking the time to undertake gentle stretching exercises each day is a good way of maintaining muscle and joint flexibility.**

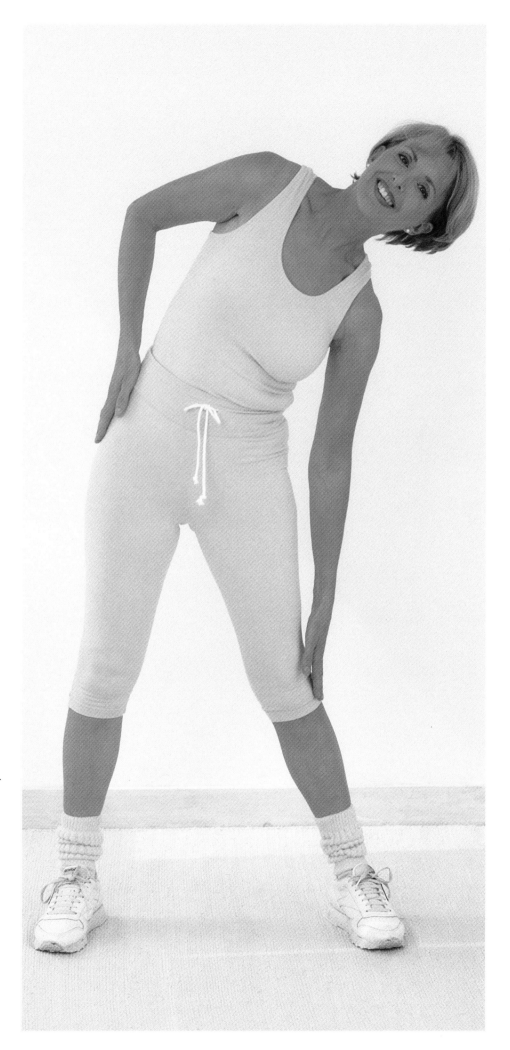

The harmful effects of free radicals

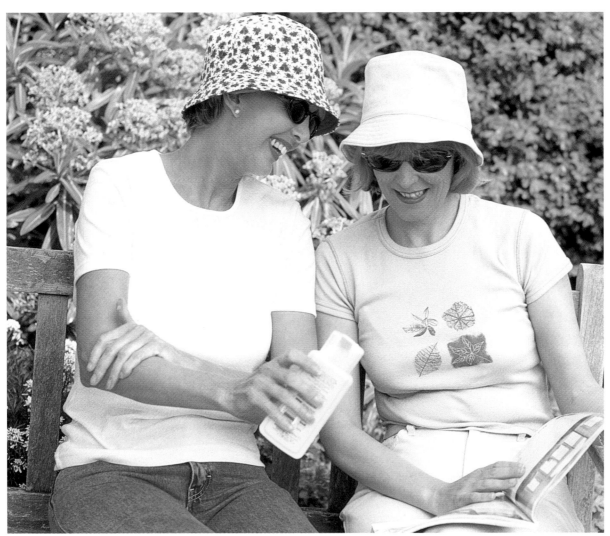

Although the causes of aging are not entirely understood, we now know that damage to the body by substances known as free radicals plays a critical role. In fact, doctors and nutritionists say that, without doubt, the most important fight against aging should be against free radical damage. Although free radicals have received much press attention, few of us understand exactly what they are or how they affect the body.

free radicals

Oxygen is essential for life, but it can also be considered a poison. This is because when oxygen is used for essential processes inside the body, it leads to the production of damaging molecules known as free radicals. The most damaging characteristic of free radicals is their chemical structure in that they contain an unpaired electron. This means that they roam around the body "searching" for healthy molecules to pair with. Unfortunately, this pairing process damages the host molecule and irreversibly changes the DNA (material that carries genetic information). If free radicals are allowed to damage body cells in this way over a long period of time, the result is extensive cell damage and aging, as well as diseases such as arthritis, heart disease, cataracts and cancer.

A good way to understand free radical damage to the body is to think of it as continuous internal radiation. Yet free radicals are not just created by normal bodily processes; they are also created by oxidation outside the body. For example, combustion processes, radiation from the sun, cigarette smoking and environmental pollution all give rise to free radicals. Also, some foods and drinks (fried food and alcohol, for example) generate more free radicals than others.

the fight against free radicals

Although our bodies have evolved their own defences against free radicals, it is essential that we minimize exposure to free radicals where possible. This means giving up cigarette smoking (and avoiding other people's cigarette smoke), not eating burnt food, staying out of direct sunlight, not drinking too much alcohol and minimizing exposure to environmental pollution such as traffic fumes. It is also believed that sleep deprivation can increase free radical damage to the body, so we need to make sure we have sufficient sleep every night.

the best weapons: antioxidants

By far the best weapons in the war against free radicals are antioxidants, which are found in vitamins A, C and E, in co-enzyme Q10 and betacarotene, as well as in minerals such as selenium and zinc.

When free radicals are roaming around the body, antioxidant molecules can pair with them, preventing them from attacking healthy molecules. When antioxidants pair with (or "mop up") roaming free radicals they can then be eliminated from the body via the excretory systems. This way, no damage is done to the body.

One way to understand the action of antioxidants is to observe what happens when lemon juice is dropped onto the cut surface of an apple. As soon as the apple is cut and exposed to the air it reacts with oxygen and starts to discolour. Yet if lemon juice is squeezed onto the cut surface, the antioxidant action of the vitamin C in the juice will prevent the discoloration. However, this protection is only temporary and the cut surfaces will start to oxidize as the antioxidant function wears down.

The importance of antioxidants in your diet cannot be over-estimated. It is crucial for everyone, especially older people, to eat foods rich in antioxidant vitamins and minerals. Nutritionists recommend eating plenty of fresh fruit and vegetables on a daily basis. Antioxidants are also available in the form of supplements.

▽ The darker outer leaves of lettuce contain betacarotene, an antioxidant thought to protect against some cancers.

△ Strawberries contain a phytochemical called ellagic acid which is believed to fight against cancer.

Where to find antioxidants

The main antioxidant nutrients are vitamins A, C, and E, zinc and selenium. Foods containing these vitamins and minerals should be part of your daily diet. In addition to these vitamins and minerals, there are other substances known as phytochemicals, found in plants, that also have antioxidant properties. These include bioflavanoids (found in citrus fruit) and lycopene (found in tomatoes). Some amino acids, such as cysteine and glutamic acid also have antioxidant effects. Cysteine and glutamic acid are found in white meat, tuna, lentils, beans, nuts, seeds, onions and garlic.

The following foods are excellent sources of antioxidants and can be eaten in abundance:

- Sweet potatoes
- Carrots
- Watercress
- Broccoli
- Peas
- Cauliflower
- Tomatoes
- Citrus fruit
- Watermelon
- Strawberries
- Seeds
- Nuts

Anti-aging Diet

Through the leaps made in the science of
nutrition, we now know that the food we eat
can make a huge contribution to our health
and wellbeing. We can help prevent many
aging-related problems, such as heart disease,
by concentrating on some food groups in the
diet and limiting others.

Revising your eating habits

Between the ages of 40 and 65, life becomes more sedentary for many of us. We may retire and have fewer personal obligations than before. A slower lifestyle means that the body needs fewer calories. Yet our vitamin and mineral requirements remain the same or increase in order to prevent cell aging and dietary deficiencies.

healthy eating patterns

Since diet is so important as you get older, it is advisable to periodically alter your diet and eating patterns. Do you eat with health in mind or are your eating habits based on convenience? Are you prone to eating lots of "empty calories" in the form of fatty and sugary foods? Are you at risk of diet-related health problems such as osteoporosis (a chronic disease that weakens the bones)?

Nutritionists recommend a low-fat diet based on fresh fruit and vegetables, unrefined, complex carbohydrates and protein foods such as oily fish. This keeps the immune system in good working order and helps to prevent cell aging and degenerative diseases caused by free radicals (highly reactive molecules within our bodies). The World Cancer Research Fund estimates that 40 per cent of cancers (approximately 4 million cases worldwide) can be avoided by following a healthy diet and not smoking.

▷ **Avoid elasticated waist bands on skirts and trousers since they allow clothes to remain comfortable, instead of giving early warning of creeping weight gain.**

◁ **White pasta offers less fibre, minerals and vitamins than wholemeal pasta, but is still a useful source of low-fat complex carbohydrate.**

do you need to lose weight?

Excessive weight gain is not inevitable as we age. In fact we should not weigh more than 9 kg/20 lbs more at the age of 50 than we did at 20, regardless of height. Many wieght charts are standardized to include age, height and sex; if your weight is 20 per cent above or below the standard, it is advisable to have a medical check up to ensure no problems exist.

In 1999, Dr Margaret Ashwell, a nutritionist, recommended a new and simple method of determining acceptable weight to the British Royal Society of Medicine. According to her method, if your waist measurement is less than half your height measurement, then your weight does not present a health hazard. If this method is applied to people in the UK, 15 per cent of men and 11 per cent of women can be considered dangerously overweight.

Another way of assessing weight is to calculate what percentage of your body consists of fat. This is a test that can be performed by some health centres and sports clinics. On average our bodies are composed of approximately: 63 per cent water, 22 per cent protein, 13 per cent fat and 2 per cent vitamins and minerals.

If your fat ratio is significantly higher than 13 per cent a doctor is likely to advise you to reduce your fat intake and increase the amount of aerobic exercise you do. These are important measures in the prevention of chronic health problems.

As you get older it is advisable to avoid foods that contain too many additives such as sugar and salt, which are implicated in health problems such as hypertension and diabetes. As part of your dietary reassessment, study the labels of the foods in your kitchen. Compare the additives and ingredients in different foods. Ideally, the food on your shelves should be low in calories, saturated fat, sodium and sugar, and high in fibre and vitamins and minerals. If you become familiar with the composition of different foods, you will quickly become adept at monitoring what you are eating.

Throw away unhealthy recipes
When you are revising your eating habits, it can help to throw away recipes for unhealthy foods such as cakes, puddings and rich dishes that contain a lot of cream. This way you will not be tempted to cook them. Start to build a collection of new recipes that are low in fat and high in fibre, vitamins and minerals. Buy yourself a new cookery book containing healthy recipes.

▷ **Keep a variety of easy-to-prepare raw fruit and vegetables as nibbles, and only buy cakes and biscuits for special occasions.**

▽ **Try to make time to sit down and enjoy meals, rather than grabbing a quick snack on the run.**

How to eat a healthy diet

What we eat, and when, has a direct effect upon our body systems. By eating a balanced diet we can stay healthy, maintain energy levels, preserve healthy muscles and bones and help our brains to work efficiently, no matter how old we are. The guidelines for a balanced diet are straightforward and are based on eating the right amounts of foods from various different food groups.

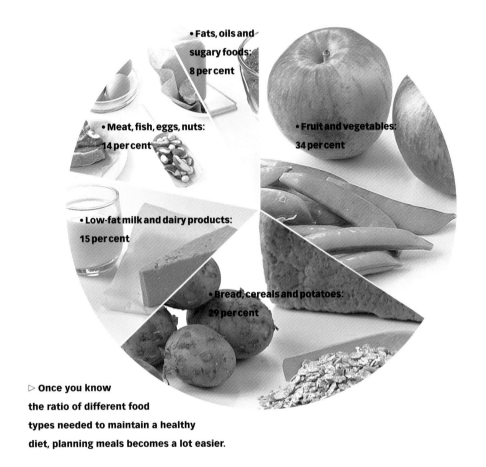

- Fats, oils and sugary foods: 8 per cent
- Meat, fish, eggs, nuts: 14 per cent
- Fruit and vegetables: 34 per cent
- Low-fat milk and dairy products: 15 per cent
- Bread, cereals and potatoes: 29 per cent

▷ **Once you know the ratio of different food types needed to maintain a healthy diet, planning meals becomes a lot easier.**

food groups

There is a broad consensus among doctors and nutritionists that foods fall into several discrete categories and that we should eat specific percentages of different types of foods. The breakdown of these food groups is shown in the pie chart above.

This breakdown exists as a rough guide and is not designed to be followed on a rigid daily basis. It does, however, show the emphasis that should be placed upon fruit, vegetables and complex carbohydrates.

when to eat

Traditionally, people have eaten three meals a day: breakfast in the morning, lunch at midday and dinner in the evening. Although this is a useful template, people often develop the habit of eating a small breakfast and lunch, and a large evening meal. This has a detrimental effect on digestion, especially as our digestive systems become more

sluggish with age. It also means that we have an inadequate supply of energy at the times of day when we are most active and a calorie overload at the end of the day when we are winding down.

A preferable eating pattern is a large breakfast, a substantial lunch and a comparatively small meal early in the evening. Alternatively, some people favour the grazing approach to eating in which they eat small quantities of food throughout the day. This prevents overloading the

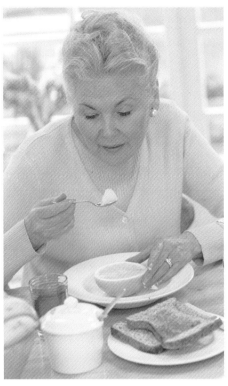

△ **Allow yourself time to enjoy a healthy breakfast each morning.**

digestive system and ensures a consistent supply of energy throughout the day. The grazing method is also a good way of stabilizing blood sugar levels in the body, which may be useful for people suffering from adult-onset diabetes.

how healthy is meat?

Meat has had a lot of bad press in many countries in recent years for reasons such as infection with bovine spongiform encephalopathy (BSE) or the presence of antibiotics. Meat is high in saturated fat, which is implicated in the development of heart disease. It is also high in an amino acid called arachidonic acid, which increases levels of pro-inflammatory chemicals and should therefore be avoided by people of a rheumatic disposition. It does, however, still remain possible to eat meat safely. If you are concerned about the presence of antibiotics, choose organically produced meat, and cut away any visible fat on meat to avoid consuming too much saturated fat. Moderation is the key: the World Cancer Research Fund recommends that no more than 75g/3oz of meat should be eaten per day.

Eaten in moderation, meat is a useful source of antioxidant minerals such as zinc and selenium. Antioxidants can help prevent degenerative diseases, such as cancer. Beef is a good source of iron, zinc and B vitamins; choose lean cuts such as topside in which the fat content is only 2.7 per cent per 115g/4oz – minced beef can contain up to 25 per cent fat.

Pork supplies B vitamins, iron, zinc and selenium. Excess fat should be removed, and pork crackling should be avoided. Chicken supplies only about half the zinc and iron of red meats, but if the skin is removed prior to cooking it is very low in fat. It is also an excellent source of the antioxidant selenium.

Older people are advised to eat plenty of oily fish because they contain omega-3 fatty acids. These are essential fatty acids that are vital for health but cannot be made by the body. Omega-3 fatty acids can help to fight against heart disease, and are found in abundance in salmon, mackerel, sardines, pilchards, herrings, kippers and tuna.

◁ Buying small, easy-to-prepare cuts of meat will help you to monitor the amount of saturated fat that you eat each day.

▽ Instead of using heavy, fattening sauces to liven up fish, try sprinkling it with herbs to help bring out the full flavour.

Anti-aging foods

The general guidelines for the anti-aging diet are: keep your calorie consumption and saturated fat intake down; eat plenty of wholegrains, oily fish and fresh fruit and vegetables; and cut down on salt and sugar. In addition to these general guidelines, there are specific foods that have a role in anti-aging and that you should regularly include in your diet.

△ An avocado a is very versatile fruit that can be eaten either cooked or raw, and used in both savoury and sweet dishes.

avocado

This fruit, which is usually eaten as a vegetable, is a good source of healthy monounsaturated fat that may help to reduce levels of a bad type of cholesterol in the body. Avocado is a good source of vitamin E and can help to maintain healthy skin and prevent skin aging (vitamin E may also help alleviate menopausal hot flushes). It is rich in potassium which helps prevent fluid retention and high blood pressure.

berries

All black and blue berries such as blackberries, blueberries, blackcurrants and black grapes contain phytochemicals known as flavonoids – powerful antioxidants which help to protect the body against damage caused by free radicals and aging.

cruciferous vegetables

The family of cruciferous vegetables includes cabbage, cauliflower, broccoli, kale, turnip, brussels sprouts, radish and watercress. Cruciferous vegetables assist the body in its fight against toxins and cancer. You should try to consume at least 115g/4oz (of any one or a combination) of these vegetables on a daily basis. If possible, eat them raw or very lightly cooked so that the important enzymes remain intact.

△ Blueberries are rich in vitamin C and flavonoids which help to prevent cancer.

▽ Broccoli, cabbage and cauliflower contain high levels of cancer-fighting phytochemicals.

△ You can boost your garlic consumption by taking it as a supplement.

△ Rice and pasta are good low-fat carbohydrates.

garlic

Eating a clove of garlic a day (raw or cooked) helps to protect the body against cancer and heart disease. The cardioprotective effects of garlic are well recorded. One 1994 study in Iowa, USA, of 41,837 women between the ages of 55 and 69 suggested that women who ate a clove of garlic at least once a week were 50 per cent less likely to develop colon cancer. Another study at Tasgore Medical College in India suggested that garlic reduced cholesterol levels and assisted blood thinning more effectively than aspirin, thus helping to reduce the risk of heart disease.

ginger

This spicy root can boost the digestive and circulatory systems, which can be useful for older people. Ginger may also help to alleviate rheumatic aches and pains.

▽ A glass of hot water with a little ginger can alleviate nausea, especially car and sea sickness.

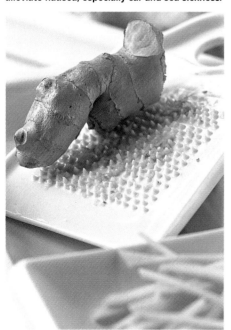

nuts

Most varieties of nuts are good sources of minerals, particularly walnuts and brazil nuts. Walnuts, although high in calories, are rich in potassium, magnesium, iron, zinc, copper and selenium. Adding nuts to your diet (sprinkle them on salads and desserts) can enhance the functioning of your digestive and immune systems, improve your skin and help prevent cancer. Nuts may also help control cholesterol levels. Never eat rancid nuts, however, as they have been linked to a high incidence of free radicals.

△ Brazil nuts are rich in magnesium and selenium.

soya

Menopausal women might find that soya helps to maintain oestrogen levels. Soya may alleviate menopausal hot flushes and protect against Alzheimer's disease, osteoporosis and heart disease. Look out for fermented soya products, which are more easily digested, therefore more nutritional, and do not generally cause food intolerances. You may want to check that soya products have not been genetically modified. Soya should not be confused with soy sauce, which is full of salt and should be used sparingly, if at all.

▷ Chilled water melon is refreshing on hot days.

wholemeal pasta and rice

Complex carbohydrates provide a consistent supply of energy throughout the day and should make up the bulk of your diet. Wholemeal pasta is an excellent complex carbohydrate. It is high in fibre and contains twice the amount of iron as normal pasta. Brown rice is another recommended complex carbohydrate, which is high in fibre and B vitamins.

watermelon

Both the flesh and seeds of the watermelon are nutritious so try blending them together in a food processor and drinking as a juice. The flesh contains vitamins A, B and C; the seeds contain selenium, essential fats, zinc and vitamin E, all of which help against free radical damage and aging.

Food intolerance

Many people find that they start to suffer from food intolerance as they grow older. This is partly due to long-term exposure to an irritating substance and partly due to the fact that the digestive system becomes less efficient with age. Eating foods to which you are intolerant is like continually stubbing your toe – the discomfort will become worse over a period of time and eventually the damage can become permanent.

what is food intolerance?

A food intolerance should not be confused with an allergy. An intolerance occurs when the body finds a substance difficult to cope with, whereas an allergy to a substance is an active fight that involves the body's immune system.

Although there are many different types of food intolerance, some foods are more likely to cause intolerances than others. They include soya products, caffeine, chocolate, orange juice, tomatoes and food additives. Two foods that commonly cause intolerances are cow's milk and wheat (or other grains).

If you have an intolerance to cow's milk, this means that your body finds it difficult to digest lactose, the sugar found in milk. As a result, lactose moves through the

△ Tomatoes are a good source of disease-fighting antioxidants, but some people may find they develop an intolerance to them.

◁ By keeping a diary of foods ingested each day, it is often possible to detect small intolerances before they become too problematic.

intestines undigested and when it reaches the colon, bacteria start to ferment it, producing gas. The result may be abdominal discomfort, flatulence and diarrhoea.

An intolerance to wheat and grains means that you have difficulty digesting the protein gluten. Gluten intolerance can cause weight loss, loss of appetite, abdominal cramps and poor vitamin and mineral absorption from food.

detecting food intolerances

You may already suspect that you have an intolerance to a particular food, simply because you suffer discomfort when you consume it. To confirm that this is the case, try eliminating the suspicious food for a month before re-introducing it to your diet. Keep a daily diary of your symptoms and note whether they return when you re-introduce the food. Alternatively, you can seek the professional advice of a doctor, dietician or naturopath.

▷ Soya milk offers a good alternative to dairy products containing lactose. Although soya beans have a higher fat content than other pulses, the fat is mostly unsaturated and is considered to be non-harmful.

dealing with food intolerances

There is no cure for food intolerance except simply avoiding the relevant foods. If you identify the foods that you cannot tolerate, you can look for alternatives that satisfy your nutritional needs and personal tastes. For example, if you cannot tolerate orange juice, drink

Signs to look out for

You may have a food intolerance if you suffer from any of the following symptoms on a regular basis:

- Anxiety
- Depression
- Fatigue
- Headaches
- Skin disorders
- Asthma
- Joint or muscle pain
- Rheumatoid arthritis
- Ulcers (mouth or stomach)
- Water retention
- Stomach bloating
- Nausea
- Vomiting
- Constipation
- Diarrhoea
- Irritable bowel syndrome

▽ For those suffering from lactose intolerance, live yogurt is easier to digest than milk, and is a good way to boost calcium levels.

apple juice instead. It may not even be necessary to exclude foods completely. For example, if you have an intolerance to cow's milk you may still be able to tolerate a small amount of milk in one cup of tea a day.

If you are lactose intolerant try to avoid dairy products, and check food labels for the presence of lactose. Substitute soya milk for cow's milk. Women who need to exclude dairy products should ensure that they receive

△ Corn is a good alternative to wheat for those with a gluten intolerance.

enough calcium from other sources to maintain healthy bones. Live yogurt is a good calcium source for people who are lactose intolerant (the bacteria present in the yogurt helps to break down lactose). Gluten intolerant people should avoid wheat, rye, and barley. Switching to corn, rice, soya, and potato starch can be helpful.

Warning

If you are suffering from unusual digestive complaints such as nausea, diarrhoea or persistent indigestion, seek a diagnosis from your doctor before you make any dietary changes. A full elimination diet should be supervised by a medical professional.

Dietary tips

Nutritionists and dietary therapists have now identified the eating habits that bring health and those that do not. The main guideline for a healthy diet as we grow older is to eat a diet rich in antioxidants – substances that actively fight the cell damage that leads to aging. Antioxidants are found in abundance in fruit and vegetables. There are a number of other guidelines that become especially important with age.

good and bad fats

Some fats are necessary for health and others are harmful. Unsaturated fats are essential to our bodies for the transportation of vitamins A, D, E and K, lowering harmful cholesterol, and aiding the nervous system, cardiovascular system and brain. Good sources of unsaturated fat are olive oil, oily fish, nuts and seeds.

Saturated fats are linked to the build up of fatty deposits on artery walls leading to blocked arteries. There may also be an association between high saturated fat intake and certain cancers. Foods that contain saturated fat should be avoided or eaten in moderation. They include meat,

△ **Stir frying is a quick and easy way to prepare appetizing low-fat meals**.

dairy products and palm and coconut oils. Fried food and fat found in cakes, cookies and prepared meals should also be avoided.

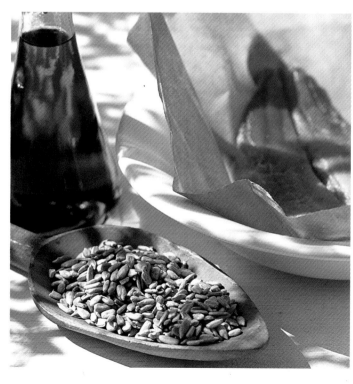

▷ **Sunflower seeds are a good source of vitamin B$_3$ (niacin) which can fight against depression, circulatory problems, high blood pressure and cholesterol, tinnitus, and breathing problems in asthmatics.**

Avoiding fats
- Check food labels for hidden fats.
- Choose low-fat cooking techniques, such as grilling or stir-frying.
- When cooking meat, place it on a rack so that excess fat drips off.
- Add yogurt rather than cream to your desserts.
- Buy canned fish in brine rather than in oil.

understanding cholesterol

Not all cholesterol is unhealthy. There are two types of cholesterol: high density lipoprotein (HDL) which is popularly known as "good cholesterol", and low density lipoprotein (LDL), popularly known as "bad cholesterol".

Explained simply, HDL stops the build up of fatty deposits in the arteries and LDL creates them. If your HDL levels are high compared to your LDL levels, then you are at a low risk of cardiovascular disease. The ideal ratio is thought to be three parts HDL to one part LDL.

As you age it is important to maximize your cardiovascular health by keeping your LDL levels low and your HDL levels high. The best way to achieve this is to avoid fried foods and saturated and hydrogenated fats – the main sources of LDL. (Hydrogenation is a process that turns vegetable oil into hard fat.) Other ways to promote a healthy HDL/LDL balance include:
- eating plenty of garlic
- a diet rich in vitamin C
- eating foods rich in vitamin B$_3$
- including plenty of oily fish in your diet

cut out sugar and salt

Although complex carbohydrates, such as whole grains and pulses, are good for us, simple carbohydrates such as refined sugar are not. All forms of sugar whether brown sugar, white sugar, honey or syrup cause our blood sugar levels to increase rapidly. If this instant supply of energy is not used, the body stores it and eventually it is converted into fat. Keep refined sugar intake to a minimum; it has no nutritional value and causes sudden highs in blood sugar levels, followed by slumps that can leave you feeling moody and irritable. If you have a sugar craving, eat a piece of fruit. Sugar, and the foods that it is found in (candy, cakes and many other processed foods), are said to contain "empty calories" because they offer short-lived energy without the benefit of nutrients such as vitamins and minerals.

Cut down on salt or eliminate it from your diet and never eat more than about a teaspoon a day. Too much salt causes fluid retention, places stress on the kidneys and heart, and lessens the amount of potassium absorbed by the body. High blood pressure becomes more likely as we get older, and a high-salt diet can contribute to its development. Check for the presence of salt or sodium chloride on food labels, and where possible avoid adding salt to food during cooking or at the dining table.

fibre – nature's broom

Dietary fibre is essential for a healthy digestive system. It is sometimes referred to as "nature's broom" because it sweeps

△ **The membranes around orange segments contain a soluble fibre, pectin, which helps to lower levels of LDL cholesterol. Oranges also contain vitamin C and flavonoids, which maintain healthy skin and help in the fight against disease.**

through the intestines transporting debris and residue out of the body. Fibre is not digested by the body so it retains its original mass and contributes to healthy, regular bowel movements. It may also decrease the amount of fat absorbed by the body and help to protect the arteries. Fibre absorbs water in the intestines so it is important to drink extra water if you include a lot of fibre in your diet. Try to eat plenty of natural sources of fibre such as lentils, dried beans, seeds, whole grains, fruit and vegetables.

be sparing with protein

Protein is essential for life, but only a very small amount is needed each day. Too much can contribute to a variety of health problems, including osteoporosis. Most of us eat far more protein than we actually need and, contrary to popular belief, many plant foods are rich in protein. For example, a meal containing rice and lentils, but no meat or dairy products, is a source of good quality protein. Estimates for protein requirement vary, but range from 4.5 to 8 per cent of our total calorie intake. Try to eat less protein foods and replace animal proteins with plant proteins, such as tofu, spinach and pumpkin seeds. Plant proteins are advantageous in that they contain fibre but no saturated fat.

▽ **Beans offer a good source of low-fat fibre and are cholesterol free and high in protein, iron and B vitamins.**

▽ **Tofu is made from soya beans and is a valuable addition to vegan and dairy-free diets.**

Drinking fluids

Water is a vital nutrient and one that we cannot store in the body. We lose water all the time through sweat, urination, defecation and simply exhaling water vapour. It is essential to drink a minimum of 1.5 litres/$2\frac{1}{2}$ pints of water a day, preferably 2 litres/$3\frac{1}{2}$ pints. As we grow older our thirst mechanism becomes less reliable and we are more prone to dehydration.

water – the healthiest drink

The best drink to keep the body hydrated is pure water. Fruit and vegetable juice and herbal teas are also good choices. Soft drinks that contain flavouring, preservatives and sugar can place stress on the body or add "empty calories" to your diet and should be drunk infrequently. If your diet is very high in fibre, you will need to drink extra water (fibre absorbs water in the intestines).

Carbonated water is an acceptable alternative to still water, but it should be drunk in moderation, as dietary therapists believe it raises the pH of the stomach and the reduced acidity makes it harder for the body to digest protein.

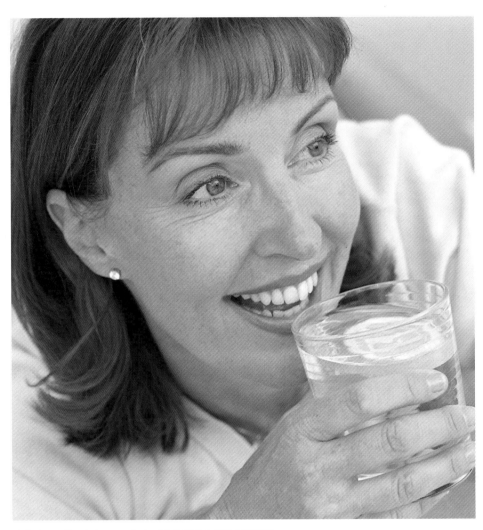

△ **A glass of body-temperature water with a slice of lemon is a good drink to wake up the body each morning.**

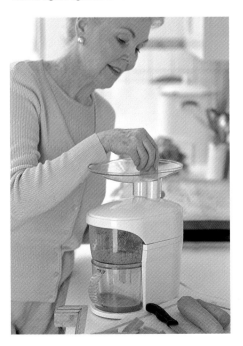

▽ **Carrot juice is a tasty source of vitamin A, which fights against cancer and heart disease.**

Apart from preventing dehydration, keeping up your fluid intake may help to prevent bladder cancer as you get older. This may be because a regular flow of fluid prevents prolonged exposure of the bladder tissue to potential carcinogens. Drinking water is also good for your appearance: if your skin is properly hydrated it will look younger and healthier.

don't rely on thirst

As you grow older you should not rely on feeling thirsty to tell you when to drink. Instead, drink water throughout the day and monitor the colour of your urine. A pale golden colour means that you are probably getting enough to drink; dark amber means that you are not. Dehydration can be exacerbated by hot climates, exercise, alcohol, illness (especially vomiting and diarrhoea) and taking diuretic medications.

Most people do not drink enough fluid on a daily basis to keep the body fully hydrated, or they drink too many diuretic drinks, such as coffee, which increase the body's fluid loss. As a result, many of us suffer from symptoms of mild dehydration such as fatigue and headaches, and the body functions at a sub-optimum level. If you become seriously dehydrated, your skin becomes dry, your eyes appear sunken, your urine turns dark and you may suffer from constipation, dizziness, nausea, cramps, confusion, low blood pressure and itchiness.

△ **The flavonoids in red grape skins are thought to reduce arterial and immune system aging.**

alcohol

As you get older, alcohol can take its toll on the body. Drinking more than recommended guidelines places stress on the liver, hinders the absorption of nutrients, dehydrates the body, damages cells and causes the body to age prematurely. This is especially noticeable in the skin. Yet if alcohol is drunk in moderation, it can offer some benefits. Half to one unit per day for women and two units for men may help to reduce arterial aging and heart attacks. Scientists are not entirely certain how alcohol produces these beneficial effects, but some believe that it may prevent fat from oxidizing and forming deposits on artery walls.

Red wine may be beneficial if drunk in moderation. The flavonoids in red grape skins are thought to have antioxidant properties. Antioxidants help to prevent disease and the degeneration of body cells.

caffeinated drinks

Some of our most popular drinks, such as tea, coffee and cola drinks, contain caffeine. Apart from its diuretic effect, opinions are mixed about whether caffeine constitutes a threat to health. It is therefore advisable to drink caffeinated drinks in moderation (no more than 2 or 3 cups a day). Overuse may cause sleep disturbances, prevent

vitamins and minerals from being used effectively by the body, raise blood pressure and cause an increase in the secretion of stress hormones. Different types of coffee contain different amounts of caffeine: instant coffee contains the least caffeine; ground, unfiltered coffee contains the most. A good alternative is steamed decaffeinated coffee, which unlike other decaffeination processes, does not involve the addition of toxic chemicals. For a healthier alternative try dandelion coffee or a cereal beverage made with barley or chicory.

How to stay hydrated

- Eat foods with a high water content such as fruit and soup.
- Drink a glass of water as soon as you get up in the morning.
- Drink a glass of water at least half-an-hour before each meal.
- Sip water at 10 to 15-minute intervals during exercise (many people underestimate how much they sweat; try weighing yourself before and after you sweat).
- Drink water at the first sign of a headache or muscle cramp.
- Choose low-caffeine or decaffeinated drinks that will not have a diuretic effect on the body.
- Buy a juicer and make your own fruit and vegetable juices. Alternatively, make fruit smoothies in a blender.

△ **Keeping the body hydrated helps to cleanse the body by ensuring the elimination of toxins.**

herbal teas

A great variety of herbal teas are available, and you can even make your own herbal infusions with medicinal benefits. Herbal teas have the benefit of hydrating the body while being caffeine free. To make a cup of camomile tea, place a handful of the fresh herb in a teapot, pour on boiling water, leave to infuse for 5 minutes, stir and pour through a strainer. Camomile can help to relieve anxiety and insomnia.

▷ **Readily available and easily prepared, mint tea is a good remedy for nausea, migraine, indigestion, flatulence, and irritable bowel syndrome.**

Weight loss

△ **A healthy alternative to oil-based salad dressings is to squeeze fresh lemon juice onto the salad immediately before serving.**

As you grow older, being overweight puts you at risk of a range of health problems including diabetes and hypertension. If you are overweight, changing your diet can significantly reduce your chances of illness (as well as raise your self-esteem). You do not have to go on a starvation diet to lose weight, but you do need to make long-term changes to your eating patterns by cutting out processed foods and full-fat products.

consume fewer calories

The rate at which you burn energy or calories – your metabolic rate – slows down as you get older (a calorie is the amount of heat needed to raise the temperature of 1 litre/ $1^3/_4$ pints of water by one degree). You may find that continuing to eat the same amount that you did previously causes you to slowly gain weight. The way to lose weight is to consume fewer calories than you expend so that the body is forced to burn stored fat.

Daily calorie requirements vary according to your lifestyle, but, as a rough guide, women need approximately 2,000 calories

per day and men need 2,500. These figures increase if you have an active lifestyle. By eating 1,000 calories less than these energy requirements each day, you should be able to achieve a steady weight loss of about 1kg/2$^1/_4$ lbs a week, although the loss may be higher at first due to fluid losses. It is not advisable to lose more than 1kg/2$^1/_4$ lbs a week as you are likely to be losing fluid, and bone and muscle mass, all of which can accelerate the aging process.

Many foods are labelled with their calorie contents, so it is easy to become familiar with the energy values of different foods. You should, however, try not to count calories obsessively.

types of food

The types of food that you should eat during a weight-loss diet are the same as those for a normal, well-balanced diet: concentrate on complex carbohydrates and fresh fruit and vegetables. Avoid fatty foods especially saturated fats (found in meat, dairy products

▽ **Always strain herbal teas prior to drinking to allow the subtle fragrance and flavour through without any bitter aftertaste from the leaves.**

△ **Rest a slice of lemon in a glass of boiling water for five minutes for a refreshing drink to enjoy at any time of day.**

and coconut and palm oils). Remember that fats contain twice as many calories as carbohydrates and proteins:

> 1g carbohydrate = 4 calories
> 1g protein = 4 calories
> 1g fat = 9 calories

As well as eating low-fat foods, try to eat little and often. Start the day with a glass of warm (body temperature) water and a slice of lemon. Eat a breakfast of wholegrains – such as wholemeal toast or muesli – half an hour after getting up. Avoid butter and use skimmed instead of full-fat milk. Snack on raw vegetables until lunch time and then make lunch the main meal of the day. Drink fruit juices, smoothies made with low-fat yogurt and herbal teas in the afternoon. Try to eat a light dinner a minimum of 3 hours before going to bed. Eat raw fruit whenever you feel hungry. Keep meals under 350 calories and allow 250 calories for drinks and snacks such as apples and carrots.

tips for losing weight

Before starting to diet, set yourself a target weight. If you are particularly overweight, you may want to decide this in conjunction

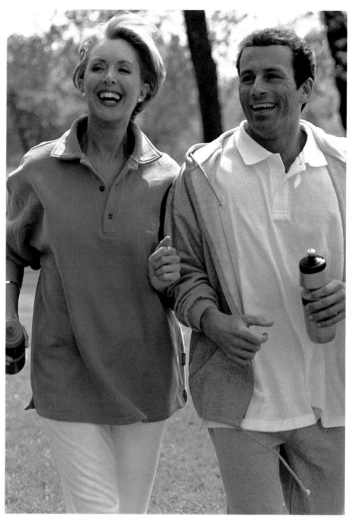

△ **Many people find exercise easier to maintain if they undertake it as a routine social interaction, such as jogging with a partner each day, or exercising the dog.**

◁ **Fluid, longline clothing is more slimming than clothing that cuts the body in half or is more bulky.**

with your doctor. If you are only slightly overweight, you may simply want to slim down until you can fit into a favourite item of clothing. If you have a lapse in your diet, do not see it as a reason to give up. Remember that you are only human.

Avoid alcohol: not only is it high in calories, but research in Holland has found that people who drank alcohol half an hour before a meal ate quicker and consumed more calories than those who remained alcohol free. Instead, drink a glass of water before a meal to help you feel full.

Avoid using dieting aids or diuretics to assist weight loss, since they will upset the body's natural balance, and can lead to problems such as vitamin deficiencies and digestive disorders.

Combine your weight-loss diet with regular aerobic exercise. This will help to speed up fat loss and develop firm muscles.

When you have reached your target weight, continue to eat sensibly. Try to keep meals to fewer than 500 calories so the body can break down each meal easily. This allows three meals of 500 calories as well as drinks and snacks of fruit.

Dietary supplements

Although the diet can provide many essential nutrients as you grow older, there are some vitamins and minerals that you may need to take in supplement form. Some dietary therapists say that the modern Western diet and lifestyle exposes people to so many nutrient "depleters" that supplements are the best way to achieve optimum nutrition.

your nutrient needs

Deficiency in fat, carbohydrate or protein is very rare in the West, but experts believe that many of us are lacking in vitamins and minerals. However, it is difficult to work out exactly which vitamins and minerals you receive in abundance and those that you may need to supplement. The best advice is to consult a naturopath or dietician who will carry out a detailed analysis of your personal nutritional needs. Both your hair and blood can be analyzed to provide information about the nutritional state of your body.

Even without professional assessment, you can make a reasonable estimate of your needs by looking at the foods you eat in your diet and examining your lifestyle and current health. For example, if your diet includes many substances, such as salt, sugar, caffeine and alcohol, that deplete the body of nutrients, then it may be advisable to take a

△ Supplements come in many forms; chelated supplements, however, contain amino acids which make them more readily absorbed by the body for maximum benefit.

multivitamin and mineral supplement. Diet can sometimes be misleading though; you may eat healthy foods but still have problems absorbing all the nutrients you need for health.

If you have a stressful lifestyle, smoke cigarettes, drink alcohol and are exposed to environmental pollution on a daily basis, then you are very unlikely to be getting all the vitamins and minerals that you need. If this is the case, taking daily supplements is probably advisable.

Your current health is often a good indication of whether you are suffering from sub-optimum nutrition or deficiency. Problems as diverse as mouth ulcers, muscle cramps, frequent colds, irritability and dry skin can often – but not always – be traced to a lack of essential vitamins and minerals.

Daily nutrient intake

Recommended daily allowances (RDAs) are standard amounts set by governments. They represent the daily amounts of a nutrient that we should consume in order to stay healthy. RDAs are criticized by some dietary therapists who say that they are far too low. It is argued that, although an RDA is high enough to prevent a deficiency disease such as scurvy (caused by insufficient vitamin C), it is not high enough to keep the body functioning at an optimum level for health and wellbeing. Critics say that RDAs should be increased to encourage people to eat healthier diets.

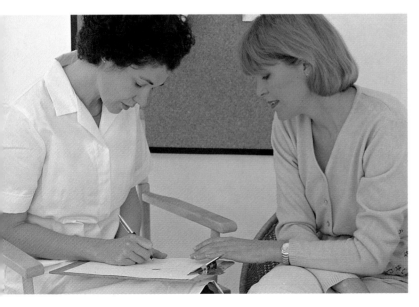

◁ Many health problems can reduce the body's ability to absorb nutrients, and it may be worth visiting a nutritionist who can advise on your dietary requirements.

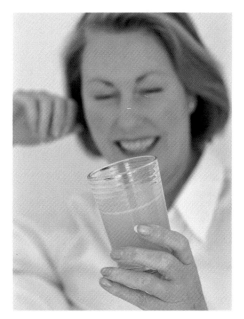

△ **Effervescent vitamin C tablets are pleasant to take, but many of them contain artificial sweeteners and flavourings.**

what are supplements?

Supplements usually come in tablet form. They contain a stated amount of the essential nutrient plus other ingredients, such as fillers, bindings and coatings to give bulk, consistency and shape to the tablet. If you cannot tolerate cow's milk, check that supplements are lactose-free. Follow the instructions regarding dosage carefully.

Some supplements (usually vitamin C and B vitamins) work on a slow-release basis because they cannot be stored efficiently by the body. To avoid the product being excreted, slow release systems gradually release the nutrients, usually over a period of six hours, to allow maximum benefit.

Liquid supplements often contain sugars and sweeteners, but are easily assimilated into the body. Always take a liquid supplement in the dosage stated and do not drink it directly from the bottle or guess the amount taken.

which supplements?

Some health problems become more common with age and they can be prevented or alleviated with supplements. Consult a nutritionist or dietary therapist if you are in any doubt which supplement to take in which dosage.

- General prevention of aging and degenerative diseases: vitamin A, C, E, betacarotene, selenium, zinc or a general antioxidant supplement.

△ **Tinctures should be dropped directly onto, or underneath, the tongue for easy absorption.**

- Menopausal symptoms: evening primrose oil, vitamin C with bioflavonoids, vitamin E, or a general multivitamin and mineral supplement.
- Prostate problems: saw palmetto (for enlarged prostate), general antioxidant supplement, or a general multivitamin and mineral supplement.
- Osteoporosis: bone mineral complex, vitamin C, or a general multivitamin and mineral supplement.
- High blood pressure: vitamin C, general antioxidant, or a general multivitamin and mineral supplement.
- Diabetes: vitamin C, B complex, zinc, chromium, or a general multivitamin and mineral supplement.
- Arthritis: vitamin C, vitamin B5, gamma-linolenic acid (GLA), eicosapentaenoic acid (EPA), bone mineral complex, general antioxidant supplement, or a general multivitamin and mineral supplement.

▽ **Gelatine capsules are unsuitable for vegetarians and vegans, who should look for seaweed alternatives.**

Staying Fit Throughout Life

In conjunction with a healthy diet, exercise is the best way to stay well, slow down the aging process and keep your body fit, toned, agile and attractive. You can reap huge benefits from relatively small increases in your activity levels. For example, walking instead of driving, swimming once or twice a week and doing some weight-lifting exercises in front of the television will quickly increase your overall fitness levels. You are never too old to start exercising.

Taking up exercise

Exercise is a vital part of preventative health care as you get older. By taking regular exercise you can prevent weight gain and keep all your organs and body systems healthy. You will also help to prevent cardiovascular disease, osteoporosis, arthritis and many other health problems.

△ T'ai chi is a non-combative martial art reputedly practised by Taoist monks in 13th-century China. It uses fluid, graceful sequences along with controlled breathing to exercise the body, calm the mind and promote self healing.

the effects of exercise

The heart is a muscle and needs to be exercised just like any other muscle in order to stay strong and healthy. Working the heart during exercise also maintains the health of the arteries and ensures that blood circulates to all the body's organs, keeping them supplied with oxygen and nutrients.

Exercise has a beneficial effect on every part of the body. It keeps the skin and hair in good condition, it makes you more energetic, it speeds up the passage of food through the digestive system, it speeds up metabolism (the rate at which the body

Staying motivated

Enthusiasm and motivation may be high at the beginning of a new exercise campaign but typically wane as the weeks go by.

- Try to make exercising part of your normal everyday routine, like combing your hair or eating dinner.
- Make exercise sociable and enjoyable: exercise with a friend or in a group.
- Choose an exercise that's right for you. If you find the gym boring, try other forms of exercise: join an exercise class, play tennis or squash or go swimming.
- A sense of achievement can act as a motivating force. Whenever you reach a target, however small, set yourself a new one.
- Fit exercise into your day. If you are very busy, find opportunities for exercise in your existing schedule. For example, cycle to work, take the stairs instead of the elevator or use a manual lawnmower to mow the grass.
- Keep reminding yourself of the health benefits of exercise and the dangers of a sedentary life. Exercise is an investment in your current and future health.

△ Touching your toes is a good way to improve flexibility in the hips and spine.

burns calories), it strengthens bones and muscles, it stabilizes blood sugar, it prevents weight gain and, if you are carrying surplus fat, it helps you to shed it. In other words, exercise prevents many of the physical changes that come with age. Exercise also has a positive effect on the mind and

△ Gardening is a great way to keep your body in good shape while enjoying the outdoors.

emotions. It is an excellent way of alleviating stress, beating depression and raising your self-esteem.

how fit are you?

Your resting heart rate provides a rough guide to your overall level of fitness. Generally, the lower your heart rate, the fitter you are. If you know that you are very unfit, you have not exercised for many years, you are overweight or you have health problems, you should consult your doctor before taking up exercise. To measure your heart rate, press your first two fingers

Fitness levels indicated by heart beats per minute

MEN

Age 20–29
Very fit: less than 60
Fit: 60–69
Moderate: 70–85
Unfit: over 85

Age 30–39
Very fit: less than 64
Fit: 64–71
Moderate: 72–85
Unfit: over 85

Age 40–49
Very fit: less than 65
Fit: 65–73
Moderate: 74–90
Unfit: over 90

Age 50 +
Very fit: less than 68
Fit: 68–75
Moderate: 76–90
Unfit: over 90

WOMEN

Age 20–29
Very fit: less than 72
Fit: 72–77
Moderate: 78–95
Unfit: over 95

Age 30–39
Very fit: less than 72
Fit: 72–79
Moderate: 80–97
Unfit: over 97

Age 40–49
Very fit: less than 75
Fit: 75–79
Moderate: 80–98
Unfit: over 98

Age 50+
Very fit: less than 75
Fit: 75–85
Moderate: 85–102
Unfit: over 102

△ **To calculate your pulse rate place the tips of your first two fingers on the pulse point at the side of your neck or on your inner wrist.**

lightly on the pulse point in your neck and count the number of beats over a 15 second period, then multiply that number by 4 to calculate the number of beats per minute.

how hard should I exercise?

While you are exercising, your optimum heart rate should always be between 60 and 80 per cent of the maximum heart rate (MHR) for your age. In order to calculate your MHR, you simply subtract your age from 220.

$$220 - age = MHR$$

Next you should calculate 60 per cent of your MHR. This is the minimum elevation of your heart rate that you should aim for during exercise. Then calculate 80 per cent of your MHR. This is the maximum elevation of your heart rate that you should aim for during exercise. A heart rate that is between 60 per cent and 80 per cent of your MHR is said to be in your "training zone". If you are 50 years old, your MHR is 170, your minimum training heart rate is 102 and your maximum training heart rate is 136. If you stick to these guidelines, you will be able to burn body fat and exercise your cardiovascular system safely.

When you have finished exercising, you should check that your heart returns to its normal rate within 10 minutes. If it takes

◁ **Once you become more agile through exercise you could try out an adventurous new sport.**

longer than 10 minutes, it is advisable that you exercise at a slower pace until you become fitter. Another quick test to ascertain whether you are exerting yourself too hard is known as the "talking test". Make sure that you can always hold a conversation while you are exercising. If you find that you are too out of breath or fatigued to talk, then you are probably exercising too hard.

▽ **Yoga tones muscles and stretches the spine.**

The benefits of exercise

There are three broad categories of exercise: aerobic exercise, anaerobic exercise and flexibility exercise. These are also known as the three "Ss": stamina, strength and suppleness. As you grow older, your heart needs a regular aerobic workout to function efficiently, your muscles need strength training to prevent them from losing mass, and your joints need flexibility exercise to maintain a full range of movement.

aerobic exercise

Aerobic exercises are those which bring your heart rate into the "training zone" (60 to 80 per cent of your maximum heart rate) and increase the body's circulation and respiratory rate. Aerobic exercise is sustained by oxygen and it is sometimes called fat-burning exercise, cardiovascular exercise or cardiowork. Aerobic exercise can be kept up for long periods of time; in fact the longer you exercise for, the greater the health benefits.

▽ **For those without joint problems, cycling provides an enjoyable form of aerobic exercise as well as a pollutant-free form of transport.**

benefits of aerobic exercise

Aerobic exercise gives the heart a good workout, burns up fat, boosts the immune system and helps to prevent the build-up of fatty deposits in the arteries. It enhances joint and muscle flexibility, stamina, sleep and digestion, and it normalizes hormone levels, helping to alleviate premenstrual syndrome and menopausal symptoms. Aerobic exercise that is also weight-bearing can help to prevent osteoporosis by strengthening and slowing down the loss of calcium in the bones.

types of aerobic exercise

Walking, jogging, cycling, swimming and dancing are effective, cheap and fun ways of taking aerobic exercise. Most gyms hold a range of classes that teach aerobic routines. Some classes use steps and weights, some are high impact and others are low impact – choose a class that matches your fitness level.

Swimming is not a weight-bearing exercise and should be combined with another form of exercise, such as walking, in order to preserve healthy bones.

getting started

Aerobic exercise can put stress on the heart if you are not accustomed to it and this is especially true for older people or those who are overweight. For this reason, it is essential to start slowly and build up gradually. As the fitness level of the body increases, the heart will slowly gain strength, until it reaches a point at which it does not need to work so hard to supply the body with sufficient oxygen to maintain exercise. At this point you will have made a positive change to your fitness levels and should start feeling the benefits of exercise.

Walking is a good way to get started on a programme of aerobic exercise: try walking to work or to the shops and walking upstairs whenever possible. As you become fitter, increase the challenge by walking faster and

△ **Walking helps to stabilize blood sugar levels, thus regulating mood swings and energy levels, as well as fighting osteoporosis, weight gain, and heart disease.**

for longer periods, or try hill-walking. You can also join a low-impact aerobic class and work at your own pace. Cardiovascular equipment in gyms – such as treadmills and training bikes – is useful because it provides immediate feedback on your heart rate, allowing you to slow down if you are working too hard. Once you have reached a reasonable level of fitness, try to do at least 35 minutes of aerobic exercise (excluding warming up and cooling down) three or four times a week.

anaerobic exercise

The term "anaerobic" means "without oxygen". During anaerobic exercise, muscles work at high intensity for a short period of time. Whereas oxygen enables long periods of exercise, anaerobic exercise is necessarily short in duration.

Anaerobic exercise results in the build up of a by-product known as lactic acid in the muscles. This causes discomfort and fatigue,

△ Regular use of arm lifts using hand weights will quickly show favourable results.

which is another reason why anaerobic exercise cannot be sustained over long periods of time. Lactic acid must leave the muscles before you can attempt further anaerobic exercise.

benefits of taking anaerobic exercise

Anaerobic exercise has far-reaching benefits for your body and health. It will keep your muscles strong and prepare your body for quick bursts of activity, such as running to catch a train or fleeing from danger. Strong, toned muscles have a variety of health benefits. They improve your

posture, they give the body a lean and taut appearance, they make you physically stronger and more powerful, and the more muscle tissue you build up, the more calories you will burn off, even during periods of complete inactivity.

You lose muscle tissue as you age (up to a third by the age of 65). In fact, a significant cause of low energy levels, fatigue and immobility in middle and later life is the decline in the amount of skeletal muscle. You can reverse this by taking anaerobic exercise several times a week.

types of anaerobic exercise

Examples of anaerobic exercise include weight lifting, sprinting, or any rapid burst of hard exercise. For example, squash is an anaerobic form of exercise because it involves short and intensive movements.

getting started

There are several ways to get started on a regular programme of anaerobic exercise. Some people join a gym and use the weights and resistance machines; others take up swimming, squash or yoga. However, the easiest (and cheapest) way to get started is to lift some weights at home.

Remember, your first aim is to tone muscles, not increase their bulk. Start by lifting a small weight a few times and increase the weight and amount of repetitions when the exercises become easier.

You can also strengthen the muscles without using weights. The simplest muscle exercises involve repeatedly clenching and

relaxing muscles. This works best on muscles such as the buttocks that are easy to isolate. It is also the principle underlying Kegel exercises which strengthen the pubococcygeal muscles and help to support the pelvic organs. To practise Kegel exercises, simply contract the pelvic floor muscles, hold for 5 seconds and release. Repeat three times.

Flexibility exercise

Practising flexibility exercises on a regular basis helps to preserve the full range of motion in the joints, improves posture and helps to alleviate problems such as arthritis. Flexibility exercises are essentially stretching exercises, such as those performed in yoga and Pilates.

Guidelines for exercising

- Stop exercising at any time if you feel dizzy, faint, nauseous or in pain.
- Always warm up and cool down before and after exercise to allow a slow build up to your training zone heart rate and to avoid injury to muscles, tendons and ligaments.
- If you lift weights, do not train the same muscle groups on consecutive days. Allow at least one or two days of rest between training sessions.
- Always pay careful attention to your posture when lifting weights.
- Try to take moderate exercise three or four times a week rather than intensive exercise intermittently.
- If possible, get a personally tailored exercise programme from a doctor, fitness instructor or personal trainer.
- Always wear comfortable, well-fitting sneakers that cushion the feet and offer good ankle support.
- When swimming, avoid the breast stroke if you suffer from back problems.
- Take care when exercising outside. Try to avoid exercising in adverse weather conditions and do not exercise in deserted places. Wear sufficient layers (you can shed them if you need to) and make sure that you are visible to traffic.
- If you lack motivation, try exercising with a friend to encourage you along.

▷ A rowing machine can help to strengthen the spine and muscular system, but for those with back problems should only be used under supervision.

yoga and Pilates

the benefits of yoga

Yoga is a holistic system. It is based upon the believe that the physical, emotional, mental and spiritual levels of your being interact within the "energetic apsect" that is the invisible double of your physical body. This aspect has its own interconnecting pathways. The main channel passes, like a motorway, through the energetic aspect of the physical spine. Anything that influences the flow of energy through your body affects you at ever level.

Yoga is one of the best ways to keep the joints and muscles flexible as you grow older. It can also relieve problems such as stress, anxiety, depression, back pain, asthma, hormonal imbalances, insomnia and irritable bowel syndrome. Although it has been practised in India for thousands of years, yoga did not appear in the West until the 19th century, and only became popular during the 1960s.

learning yoga

In the East, yoga is perceived as a route to spiritual enlightenment. In the West, however, the emphasis tends to be on yoga as a physical discipline. Western yoga classes usually focus on physical postures, known as asanas, and breathing techniques, known as pranayama.

The best way to learn yoga is from a trained teacher or therapist who will show you how to co-ordinate your breathing with your movement and help you to align your body correctly within the postures. There are also plenty of books available to help you practise yoga at home. When practising alone, make sure that you do not push your body further than is comfortable and remember to start slowly and build your flexibility gradually; the people you see in yoga books have practised for years to become flexible.

Yoga teachers recommend practising for 30 to 60 minutes a day to gain full benefit, but many people find this difficult, and 20 minutes on a regular basis is sufficient to enhance energy and stamina levels, muscle tone, digestion, flexibility, strength and general wellbeing.

◁ **This basic yoga pose, the tree, is good for strengthening the pelvis, hip joints and shoulders.**

Types of yoga

There are many different types of yoga. The type most widely practised in the West is "Hatha" ("ha" meaning "sun" and "tha" meaning "moon") representing the balancing and harmonization of positive and negative forces, usually through breathing and postures. Hatha yoga is just one branch of yoga and within Hatha yoga there are various "sub-categories":

- Astanga Vinyasa: a fast series of challenging postures performed using synchronized breathing. This is probably the most aerobic form of yoga.
- Iyengar: alignment and precision of movement are used to enhance posture, breathing and flexibility.
- Kundalini: breathing techniques and prana ("life force") are worked on to balance the body's energy and achieve relaxation.
- Sivananda: breathing and meditation are practised to produce a feeling of calm and inner peace.

△ **The Namaste pose allows you to breathe more deeply in your upper and middle back and to build up inner strength in your open heart area.**

the benefits of Pilates

The Pilates method was devised by Joseph Pilates during the 1920s and has evolved over the years to offer both mental and physical training. It aims to increase body awareness, gently realign the body, enable efficient movement and enhance control of both body and mind.

Pilates has something to offer everyone, of whatever age or current fitness level. Although overall strength is increased, one of the main benefits of Pilates is an increase in core strength. This is a phrase that is used over and over again in connection with Pilates, and it refers to the important abdominal and back muscles at your centre that support your whole body whether moving or at rest. As these muscles are strengthened, your posture will improve and you will find it easier to do daily tasks.

If you are completely new to Pilates, you will find the exercises different from others you might have tried, although there are some overlaps with yoga. First of all, Pilates is a series of movements that flow into one another without pauses. Most conventional exercise starts and stops: you might do 12 repetitions of a move, rest, and then start up again with the next sequence. Pilates concentrates on the body as a whole, stretching some muscles, strengthening others and, by helping you to function more

▽ Start and end your Pilates sessions with a couple of minutes in the relaxation position. It will help you focus on your body, as well as making you feel relaxed and refreshed.

△ Gentle stretching and toning exercises are key to the Pilates tradition. Never push yourself too far, stop if you feel in any pain whatsoever.

effectively, reducing the risk of injury, not only while you are exercising but in everything you do.

the importance of focus

Another distinguishing feature of Pilates is that to practise it you must be totally focused and concentrated, and this concentration creates a mind-body connection. This doesn't mean that conventional exercise can be done without thought of course, but it does mean that Pilates needs all your attention and focus in order to get the best results. If you sometimes feel overwhelmed by everday problems and stresses, giving all your attention to the movements of a Pilates sequence can help to still the insistent chatter of your daily life, acting like a meditation to calm your mind and help you see things more clearly. This total concentration and

attention to alignment and detail makes Pilates quite unique and very satisfying.

The best way to learn the Pilates method is in a class taught by an experienced teacher. As with yoga, breathing is an important part of the Pilates method. Try to breathe deeply into the lower ribcage during each exercise. Pilates is a very personal experience. Listen to your body and stop if anything feels uncomfortable or causes pain. As with any new exercise routine, seek the advise of a doctor before taking it up.

Controlled breathing

Learning to breathe correctly is an essential part of Pilates training. By breathing deeply into the lower ribcage and back out, you can ensure maximum use of your lung capacity. Try to breathe slowly, softly and rythmically to avoid any feeling of dizziness from overbreathing. The increase in oxygen supply provided by correct breathing will help the body replenish itself, while the exercise involved will help increase upper body flexibility. Never hold your breath during Pilates exercises as this will increase blood pressure, and waste energy in parts of the body where it is not needed.

Looking After the Body

Many of the signs of aging are invisible because they occur inside the body and do not cause external changes. Fortunately, if we look after ourselves as we enter our 40s, 50s and 60s, by eating a healthy diet and getting plenty of exercise many age-related changes can be prevented.

The skeletal system

If you have healthy bones, the chances are that you will have an active and energetic later life. As you age, your mobility and range of movement depends largely on the health of your skeletal system. It is never too late to start looking after the health of your bones and by doing so you can help to prevent a range of problems including osteoporosis, arthritis and back pain.

osteoporosis

From your 30s onwards your bones gradually start to become thinner, less dense and more porous. This loss of bone density accelerates in women after the menopause and some go on to develop osteoporosis – a disease in which the bones are so weak that they fracture even on minor impact. Men can suffer from osteoporosis too, but it tends not to appear until much later in life.

People who have osteoporosis may have a hunched appearance resulting from compression of the vertebrae in the upper spine. They may also suffer from fractures of the wrist, hip or vertebrae. Risk factors for osteoporosis include family history, poor diet, lack of weight-bearing exercise, lack of sunlight, early menopause, smoking, high alcohol, coffee or salt intake, digestive problems, eating disorders, overuse of laxatives or commercial bran products and being underweight.

Incidences of osteoporosis are increasing dramatically in Europe and the USA. In the UK approximately 200,000 bone fractures occur as a direct result of osteoporosis each year, and of these cases 80,000 people die as a result, usually due to lung or blood complications caused by immobilization.

◁ **Light skipping can be a good exercise for muscle strength, lung capacity, circulation and joint strength, as well as weight control.**

preventing osteoporosis

The key to prevention is diet. The most important mineral for healthy bones is calcium and it is important not only to include enough calcium in the diet but also to make sure that calcium absorption and uptake into the bones is maximized.

Good sources of calcium in the diet are dairy products, almonds, brewer's yeast, parsley, globe artichokes, prunes, pumpkin seeds, cooked dried beans and cabbage. Try not to rely on high-fat dairy products such as milk and cheese to supply all your calcium needs. However, if you do drink milk, remember that calcium is absorbed more efficiently in the presence of fat, so semi-skimmed milk is preferable to skimmed milk.

Factors that hinder calcium absorption include excess protein in the diet (over 40g/1½ oz per day causes calcium to be excreted in the urine), excess caffeine

△ **Adding almonds to your diet is a tasty way to boost your intake of copper, magnesium, potassium, calcium, iron and zinc.**

△ **Sprinkle pumpkin seeds into dishes during cooking or on salads and cereals for added flavour and valuable nutrients such as zinc and iron.**

△ **Most of the vitamins and minerals in cabbage are contained in the dark outer leaves; but the inner leaves are still an excellent source of fibre.**

consumption and foods such as wheatbran, chocolate and rhubarb. Avoid these foods where possible.

Both cigarette smoking and drinking excessive amounts of alcohol can dramatically increase your risk of suffering from osteoporosis. As you grow older it is essential to quit smoking and restrict drinking to within government guidelines.

Since calcium is absorbed by the gut, it makes sense to look after your digestive system. Any form of bloating, flatulence or indigestion is a sign that the digestive system is not breaking down foods efficiently. If this is the case, consult a dietary therapist who may suggest taking digestive enzymes or going on an elimination diet to establish the cause of the problem.

If you know that you have a number of risk factors for osteoporosis, and you are a postmenopausal woman, ask your doctor about the possibility of having a bone density test and taking hormone replacement therapy (HRT). A course of HRT lasting a minimum of one year has been shown to improve bone density. You can also ask whether it is appropriate to take dietary supplements. There are some multivitamin and mineral

combinations that are specially formulated for postmenopausal women and a magnesium/calcium compound (in a 2:1 ratio) may also be of benefit. Other useful supplements may include 15mg doses of zinc citrate and 50mg doses of vitamin B complex.

Weight-bearing exercise, such as walking, has a key role to play in the prevention of osteoporosis. Try to go for a brisk 30-minute walk at least every other day.

The vinegar diet

Research at a Japanese University suggests that calcium absorption is facilitated in rats by giving them a diet rich in vinegar. Other research indicates that the amount of available calcium in chicken stock increases by 40 per cent when vinegar is added to the boiling liquid. It is thought that the acetic acid in vinegar breaks down the minerals in the bones in the stock. Dr Anthony Leeds of King's College, London suggests using vinegar as a condiment at meal times since it may enhance calcium uptake.

◁ **Large quantities of coffee are known to leach vitamins and minerals from the digestive system, increasing the risk of dietary malfunctions, and contributing to conditions such as osteoporosis.**

▷ **Nowadays vinegars come in a variety of flavours, making them an appetizing addition to many dishes.**

Maintaining skeletal health

rheumatoid arthritis

Although doctors do not know the precise cause of rheumatoid arthritis it is thought to be an auto-immune disease in which the immune system starts to attack its own tissues. The most commonly affected areas are the hands and feet, followed by the knees, wrists, neck and ankles, although the disease can affect any joint in the body. Initial symptoms may include fatigue and fever followed by stiffness and swelling in the joints. Joint pain can become so bad that it restricts movement and in severe cases, bones may fuse together, making movement in the joint impossible.

Rheumatoid arthritis affects more women than men (in a 3:1 ratio) and usually appears between the ages of 40 and 50, although it can also appear in younger people, and is often accompanied by mild anaemia.

treating the symptoms of rheumatoid arthritis

You should always receive conventional medical diagnosis and treatment for rheumatoid arthritis. Doctors may recommend immuno-suppressant drugs or, in severe cases, joint replacement.

Complementary therapies can be useful for symptom relief. Dietary therapists may recommend limiting animal fats in the diet and taking supplements such as multivitamins, vitamin B complex, vitamin C, vitamin E (except when anti-coagulant drugs are being taken), glucosamine sulphate and zinc. An elimination diet may also be recommended if it is suspected that the disease is related to a food intolerance. Joint mobility can be helped by swimming, and pain can be eased by applying gentle heat to the area.

osteoarthritis

As the joints age they become prone to osteoarthritis. The cartilage in the joint wears away and the ends of the bones may rub together and develop growths which are known as spurs. The symptoms include joint pain that is exacerbated by movement, stiffness in the morning and bony growths on the fingers.

Osteoarthritis usually affects joints that have been subjected to excessive wear and tear. It is common in weight-bearing joints that have been overused in the past. Too much kneeling, for example, may cause osteoarthritis in the knees. There is no

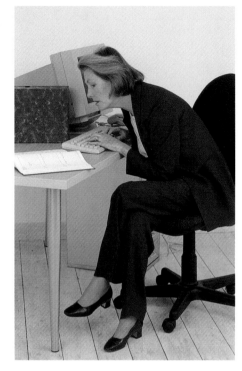

△ **This women's apalling posture is likely to lead to all sorts of health problems. When sitting you should always place both feet flat on the floor and ensure your back is straight in a chair which offers support to the small of the back.**

definitive cure for osteoarthritis; treatment consists mainly of pain relief and, occasionally, joint replacement surgery. Being overweight places unnecessary stress on the joints, so an important part of preventative care is maintaining a healthy weight or losing weight if necessary. Try to keep joints as strong and as flexible as possible by taking regular exercise. A healthy diet that is low in saturated fats, and high in fish oils may also be helpful.

supportive action for osteoarthritis

It is thought that damaging substances known as free radicals may play a major part in arthritis. Taking an antioxidant supplement can help combat free radical damage to the joints. Dietary therapists also recommend taking a daily supplement of gamma-linolenic acid (GLA). If you suffer from osteoarthritis, you should avoid tasks,

◁ **Since copper can be absorbed by the skin, many people find wearing a copper bracelet to be of use in the fight against bone disease.**

◁ **Back problems are most commonly caused by lifting heavy objects incorrectly. Always bend at the knees and hips, taking the weight on your legs rather than your spine. Keep your back straight as you lift.**

preventing back complaints

The mainstay of preventative care is regular exercise that strengthens the back muscles. Both swimming and yoga are excellent. You should also pay careful attention to your posture when sitting, standing and lying. If you work at a desk make sure that it is at a comfortable height and that your chair offers lower back support. Be careful how you lift heavy items – always bend at the hips and knees, taking the weight on your legs and keeping your back straight. Never lift and twist at the same time.

△ **Lower back pain can be relieved by lying on your back, slowly lifting your knees and clasping them towards you. If you find this difficult, try lifting and clasping just one leg at a time and slowly build up to lifting both legs.**

such as carrying heavy bags, which place unnecessary stresses and strains on the affected joints. Swim regularly and consult a physiotherapist about specific exercises to prevent muscle wasting around the affected joints. Useful complementary treatments that you may wish to try include osteopathy and chiropractic.

back problems

As you grow older, everyday stresses and strains on the spine can build up and result in chronic back problems. The people most likely to suffer are manual workers, office workers, the overweight and the elderly. Back pain is usually caused by muscle or ligament strain or disc problems.

▷ **Camomile, eucalyptus, lavender and rosemary essential oils can be used in a warm bath or hot compress to help relieve back pain.**

Easing backache

If you have back pain, there are a number of things that you can do to relieve the pain.

• Lie flat on your back with your knees bent.

• Apply a cold compress to the affected area.

• Make a hot compress, of camomile, rosemary, eucalyptus and lavender essential oils. Allow up to 8 drops of essential oil per 100ml of hot water. Soak muslin in the water and oil, squeeze out excess and apply to the back. Place a warm towel over the compress and leave for at least 2 hours. (Eucalyptus may cause skin irritation, so use sparingly.)

• Hot showers may ease pain.

• Make sure your back is adequately supported by your chair and mattress.

• Sleep on your side with your knees bent and a pillow between them (or on your back with pillows beneath your knees).

The cardiovascular system

The chances of having a heart attack or a stroke increase with age and this is something that many people fear. You can help yourself by understanding the factors that put you at risk of problems and identifying those that are preventable. For example, although you cannot change your genetic predisposition, other risk factors such as poor diet, obesity and lack of exercise are within your control.

cardiovascular disease

As we grow older we become more prone to disease of the arterial walls. Over a period of years fatty deposits build up on the inner layers of the arteries and they gradually harden into plaques known as atheroma. As a result the arteries become narrow and the flow of blood is impeded. Another age-related change that affects the arteries is a gradual thickening and loss of elasticity of the walls. In combination, these changes are known as atherosclerosis.

Damage to the arteries around the heart caused by atherosclerosis can lead to conditions such as angina, in which the blood flow to the heart is restricted. The main symptom of angina is chest pain during exertion. If blood flow to the heart is blocked, the result is a heart attack. This can be fatal or it can cause long-term damage to the heart.

A stroke happens when the brain is deprived of oxygen as a result of a blockage in a blood vessel. This causes damage to the brain, which can be fatal or cause serious impairment. Hypertension refers to abnormally high blood pressure in the arteries caused by a hardening of the walls.

preventing cardiovascular disease

Since diet and lifestyle play such a major role in cardiovascular disease it is possible to make changes that drastically reduce your chances of becoming ill. The best preventative measures are:

- Eat a low-fat, high-fibre diet that includes plenty of oily fish, fruit and vegetables (*see* Anti-aging Diet). This should become your permanent diet.
- If you are overweight, go on a weight-reduction diet. Consult your doctor about how much weight you need to lose and what types of food you should eat.
- Take aerobic exercise on a regular basis.

△ **Cook vegetables in a steamer to maintain the vitamins and minerals that are lost by boiling.**

Aerobic exercise gives your entire cardiovascular system a workout (*see* Staying Fit Throughout Life). A brisk 30-minute walk taken at least three times a week can dramatically lower the risk of premature death.

- Cut down the amount of alcohol you drink to within established guidelines.
- Reduce the amount of stress in your life. Practise relaxation techniques, particularly meditation and yoga.
- Give up smoking.
- If you are a postmenopausal woman with a history of cardiovascular disease in your family, consult your doctor about taking hormone replacement therapy (HRT).
- If you suffer from diabetes, make sure that it is meticulously controlled. Consult your doctor about this.
- You should have regular health checks, particularly cholesterol tests and blood pressure checks.

◁ **A low-fat Mediterranean diet consisting of fish, fresh fruit and vegetables, olive oil and a small amount of red wine promotes good circulation.**

△ **Aerobic exercise taken three times a week strengthens the heart and increases blood flow.**

▽ **The shoulder rise stops blood from stagnating in the lower limbs of varicose vein sufferers.**

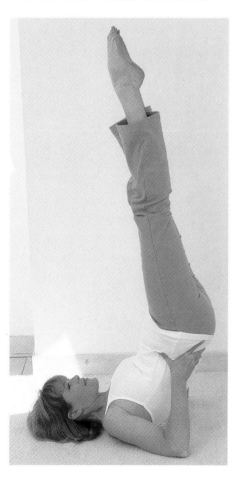

Recent research

Some dietary therapists suggest that cardiovascular disease is associated with insufficient vitamin C in the diet. Vitamin C inhibits excessive production of bad types of cholesterol that cause the build-up of fatty deposits on artery walls. It also helps to convert cholesterol into bile. A diet rich in vitamin C may help to prevent atherosclerosis. Good food sources include broccoli, peppers, watercress and citrus fruit.

varicose veins

When the valves in the veins are weakened, preventing the proper flow of blood back towards the heart, varicose veins occur. Blood then stagnates in veins, usually in the lower limbs. Varicose veins appear as swollen, twisted clusters of purple or blue veins. They are more common in women than in men, and usually worsen with age, especially during pregnancy and the menopause.

fighting varicose veins

Preventative action against varicose veins includes taking regular exercise, eating a healthy and varied diet, weight control and avoiding long periods of standing. Complementary therapies that may be useful include aromatherapy, yoga,

Giving up smoking

There is an established link between cardiovascular disease and smoking. Quitting the habit is essential in order to preserve your health. Most smokers believe that they need to smoke for a variety of psychological reasons: because it is enjoyable, relieves anxiety, boredom and stress, and aids concentration and relaxation. One of the first steps in quitting smoking is to deconstruct such myths and to recognize that the smoking is sustained by the body's physiological cravings for nicotine, which is a powerfully addictive drug. Once you have made the decision to quit smoking, set a date and seek the support of those around you. Many people successfully give up smoking by joining a support or self-help group.

△ **Citrus fruit are rich in vitamin C.**

hydrotherapy, reflexology and naturopathy. A cold compress of witch hazel may be used to ease painful varicose veins.

Folic acid is another nutrient that is implicated in cardiovascular disease. It is thought to reduce the level of an amino acid, called homocysteine, which may cause arterial clogging and heart attacks. It is suggested that eating a bowl of cereal a day may be helpful. Apart from cereal, other good sources of folic acid include spinach, peanuts, broccoli, cauliflower, asparagus and sesame seeds.

Chocolate may have hidden health benefits. Research by scientists suggests that chocolate consumption can increase blood antioxidants. Drinking cocoa in moderation may have cardioprotective properties. However, most chocolate products are also high in fat and sugar.

▽ **Research in the US and Brazil has shown that moderate chocolate consumption increases blood antioxidants within two hours of ingestion.**

The digestive system

Some people find that the digestive system becomes sluggish and less efficient with age. If your diet has always been low in fibre and high in refined foods, digestive problems may make their first appearance in middle age. Some women first experience digestive disturbances around the time of the menopause.

digestive problems

Complaints that become more common with age are indigestion, bloating, constipation, flatulence and a condition known as diverticulosis. Diverticulosis occurs when pockets form in the intestinal wall. Food can become lodged in these pockets where it ferments, producing large amounts of gas. The sufferer typically experiences flatulence, bloating and abdominal discomfort. If the pockets become infected, this gives rise to a condition known as diverticulitis. The symptoms of this are abdominal cramping, nausea and fever.

Apart from poor dietary habits, one reason why older people may suffer from digestive problems is that hydrochloric acid production declines with age. Hydrochloric acid is released from the stomach wall and it begins the breakdown of protein in the stomach. If you notice that you are prone to indigestion after eating high-protein foods, you may not be producing enough stomach acid. One solution to this is to take a digestive supplement containing betaine hydrochloride.

preventing digestive problems

The best way to prevent digestive problems is to eat a high-fibre diet. Fibre is not digested by the body so it passes through the gut intact, effectively "exercising" the intestines and adding bulk to stools. It is important to remember that if you increase the amount of fibre in your diet you should also increase the

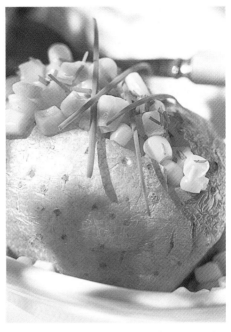

△ Baked potatoes are a good, low-fat source of dietary fibre when eaten with the skin.

amount of water that you drink. This is because fibre swells and absorbs water in the intestines.

Foods that are rich in fibre include oats, baked potatoes, lentils, brown rice, beans, fruit, wholegrain bread and wholewheat cereals. Eating cruciferous vegetables, such as broccoli and cabbage, several times a week may help to reduce the risk of colon cancer. Getting plenty of exercise is another important way of ensuring digestive health.

supportive action for digestive problems

One way of testing how well your digestive system is working is by timing how long it takes for food to pass through your system. This is known as "transit time".

To do the transit test, include a test food in your diet that you would not normally eat. It should be a food, such as beetroot, that will be visible in your stools. Alternatively, you can use charcoal tablets from a pharmacy. The time between eating the food and its first appearance in your stools should be 12–14 hours. The colour should disappear from your stools after

△ Commercial bran and laxatives should be avoided where possible. Instead eat oats, which hold water and stimulate bowel movements.

36–48 hours (this is called the retention time). If the transit time is significantly longer than 14 hours and retention time is 72 hours or more, then this is a sign that your bowel function is sluggish.

Sluggish bowel function can be treated by a wide range of complementary therapies such as massage, acupuncture, acupressure, homeopathy, herbalism and naturopathy. Naturopaths may recommend going on a cleansing diet that gives your gut a chance to clear itself. The best self-help treatment is gradually including more fibre in your diet. You should avoid taking commercial laxatives and bran products, which do not allow the body to assimilate nutrients fully, and can be harsh on the body. Specific problems may be alleviated by a number of herbal or dietary remedies.

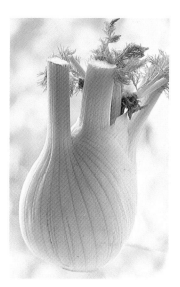

△ **Fennel can be useful in controlling flatulence.**

△ **Liquorice can help keep bowel movements regular.**

△ **Eating ginger is an excellent remedy for nausea.**

△ **Garlic and onion are good for cleansing the digestive system.**

- Garlic, peppermint, camomile and fennel may relieve flatulence.
- Linseed, prunes, rhubarb, ginger, chilli, liquorice, olive oil and honey may help to relieve mild constipation.
- Tea made with ginger root may help to alleviate nausea.
- Garlic and onions may help to cleanse the digestive system.
- Psyllium husks may help to relieve constipation. They are available in capsule form from health food shops.

▷ **Advances in dental care mean that dentures will soon be a thing of the past.**

Colon cleansing formulas are also available.
- Broad spectrum digestive enzymes, which can be bought from health food shops, may be helpful in the treatment of indigestion.
- A supplement containing acidophilus and bifidus bacteria can ensure a healthy bacterial environment in the gut.

Early warning signs

If you have any unusual or persistent digestive symptoms, such as a sudden, inexplicable change in bowel movements, blood in the stools or pain in the abdomen, consult your doctor.

Maintaining healthy teeth

The process of digestion begins in the mouth when we chew our food. Chewing has a valuable function: it increases the surface area of the food so that it is easier for enzymes to break down nutrients into their basic components. If your teeth are in poor health, they cannot perform their function properly and you will be restricted in the types of food you can eat. Pay meticulous attention to dental hygiene as you get older, visit a dentist regularly and use disclosing tablets and floss after brushing to identify and remove plaque. Gum recession, which can cause teeth to become loose in their sockets, is one of the main problems that arises with age. Try not to encourage this process: use a soft toothbrush and avoid brushing the gums.

Looking after your eyesight

The senses often become blunted with age. Changes tend to take place very gradually. If you experience a sudden change in your ability to see or hear, consult a doctor as it may be a sign of underlying illness.

vision problems

The eyes undergo a number of changes as you grow older. The lens becomes more opaque and loses its flexibility, the iris becomes sluggish, the retina can become less sensitive to light, and a condition called glaucoma – in which pressure builds up inside the eye – becomes more likely. On average, the eye of a 60-year-old person lets in half as much light as a younger person's. The most common type of age-related vision change is long-sightedness.

Warning signs of eye problems are as follows:

• difficulty seeing objects close-up (this may be caused by long sightedness)
• hazy vision, a blur around lights and the sensation of looking through fog (this may be caused by cataracts)
• loss of peripheral vision, flashes of light and floating shapes (this may be caused by retinal detachment)

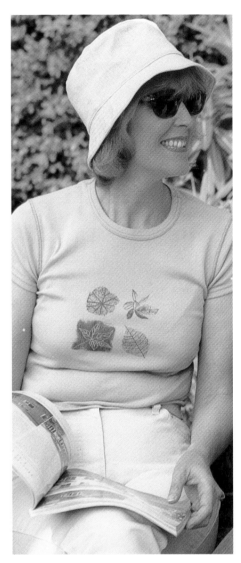

△ You should always ensure that your sunglass lenses are scratch free, otherwise they may do more harm to your eyesight than good.

• rapid or gradual vision loss and distorted vision when reading (this may be caused by macular degeneration)
• blurred vision, sudden and severe eye pain, teary, aching eyes, halos around lights, headache, nausea and vomiting (this may be caused by glaucoma).

You should have your eyesight tested yearly as you get older, and consult your doctor or ophthalmologist about any

◁ Glaucoma may occur in people over the age of 40. Nutritionists suggest a diet rich in vitamin A may be of assistance in protecting sight.

The Bates method

This is a series of eye exercises that may help to improve vision.

- splash the eyes with warm water 10 times and then cold water 10 times to increase blood circulation to the eyes.
- twice a day, rest your elbows on a table and cup your hands over your eyes. Allow yourself to relax for 10 minutes. If you do a lot of close up or computer work try to do this for one minute on a regular basis.
- try not to stare rigidly at any object for a long period of time. Every five minutes look away briefly and focus on something else for a few seconds.
- to strengthen the eye muscles, hold one index finger 10cm/4in in front of your eyes, and place the other index finger at arm's length behind it. Focus with both eyes on the nearest finger for a few seconds, blink, and then focus on the distant finger. Repeat this exercise 10 times, blinking between each change of focus to lubricate and clean the eyes.

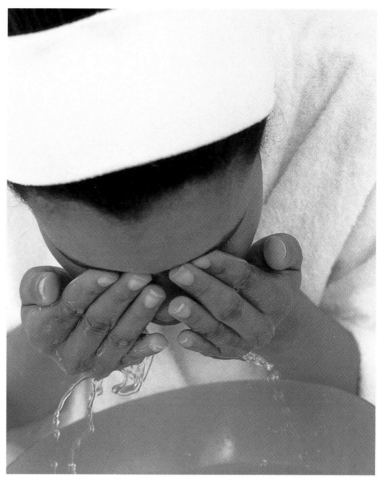

▷ **By splashing the eyes with warm and then cold water, circulation can be increased which may help against sight degeneration.**

changes in your vision. The treatment for eye problems ranges from reading glasses for long-sightedness to surgery for cataracts. If you have adult-onset diabetes, you should be particularly vigilant about having regular eye checks – diabetes is one of the main causes of blindness.

Try to protect your eyes as much as possible by not working in poor light, avoiding spending hours in front of a computer, learning some basic Bates method exercises, eating a healthy diet and taking regular exercise to increase the blood supply to the eyes. You should also wear sunglasses in bright light.

▽ **Always remove contact lenses or glasses before practising any eye exercises.**

Smell, taste and hearing

hearing problems

Problems with hearing may occur as we age due to deterioration of the sensory nerve cells and the minuscule hairs within the inner ear. Loss of hearing is a very gradual process that actually starts at the beginning of life: from the moment we are born the tiny hairs in the inner ear start to die. All of us, as we age, lose the ability to hear high-pitched sounds as clearly as when we were young. Rumbling base sounds, on the other hand, become clearer.

Age-related hearing loss is known as presbycusis. It is common in men over 40 and may be genetically influenced. Because it can be accelerated by exposure to loud noise, it is very important to avoid exposure to repetitive noise, such as music or drilling. Hearing loss is gradual and you should look out for the following warning signs:
• difficulty hearing high frequencies
• difficulty understanding speech
• difficulty hearing in noisy places
• being unable to hear sounds you used to
Consult your doctor at the first sign of hearing loss. The main treatment for age-related deafness is a hearing aid. Some people benefit from learning lip reading and sign language. Complementary treatments that may help to improve hearing include reflexology and osteopathy.

Tinnitus is another age-related problem. It presents itself as a continuous high-pitched ringing, buzzing, humming, hissing or whistling that only the sufferer can hear. There are various causes including prolonged exposure to loud noise, high blood pressure, blockage with wax, ear infection and a perforated eardrum. Some drugs cause tinnitus as a side-effect.

The best way to prevent tinnitus is to wear ear plugs in noisy situations. You should also get plenty of rest, minimize stress and limit your salt intake. Playing soft music,

▷ Consult your doctor if you begin to have difficulty following conversations.

▷**Your sense of smell may be heightened by eating zinc-rich foods such as peanuts or ginger root.**

exercising regularly, practising relaxation techniques and avoiding smoking and alcohol may ease symptoms.

smell

Our sense of smell is a much neglected asset. As well as protecting us in dangerous situations – alerting us to a fire, for example – it can also influence mood. Aromatherapists rely heavily on the olfactory system for their work. Receptors in the nose absorb smells that stimulate the olfactory bulb. Signals are then transmitted to the limbic system – part of the brain involved in the control of emotions. As you age your sense of smell is blunted and it becomes harder to differentiate between smells. Combined with a loss of taste this can mean that food becomes less appetizing

taste

There are an average of 10,000 taste buds on the tongue, the roof of the mouth, the pharynx and the oesophagus. When you are young these taste buds are replaced on a regular basis but, with age, the replacement process becomes less efficient. This means that food may not taste as interesting or diverse as it used to as you get older. Smoking, drinking alcohol and certain medications can exacerbate this. People who wear dentures may suffer additionally because the taste receptors in the palate are covered. Women may not notice any decline in their ability to taste until after menopause when oestrogen levels decline.

Although a decline in sense of taste and smell may not seem to present a serious problem, it can mean that older people start to compensate by eating different foods. For example, they may start to avoid fruit and vegetables because they taste bland, and concentrate instead on salty food, sauces and strongly flavoured cheese and meat. This can have serious implications for health. A diet with a high salt content is associated with high blood pressure, and a diet rich in saturated fat is linked to cardiovascular disease. Dietary therapists say that a decline in taste and smell may be due to a lack of zinc and that, when zinc-rich foods are eaten in the diet, taste and smell become more acute. Examples of zinc-rich food are oysters, ginger root, pecan nuts, brazil nuts, peanuts, wholewheat grains, dry split peas and egg yolk. If you want to add flavour to foods, try to use herbs and spices rather than salt.

△ **To avoid overuse of salt, try adding herbs and spices to enhance flavour.**

▽ **Pecan nuts are a source of zinc which is thought to improve taste and smell.**

Sexual health

The sexual role models that we see in the media are usually between the ages of 18 and 30. Older people are rarely depicted in a sexual way. One result of this is that we may start to feel marginalized sexually. However, most of us keep our sexual vigour as we age and many of us can look forward to staying sexually active for the rest of our lives.

age related changes

Many people enjoy sex more as they grow older because they have gained considerable sexual experience and confidence. They know what sort of sexual activities arouse them and they may feel relaxed about communicating their sexual needs and desires.

How people change in their physical responses as they age varies from person to person. Most people in their 40s do not notice any significant sexual changes. People in their 50s may begin to notice that their sexual responses are slower than before and some people may begin to suffer problems related to medication, disability or underlying illness.

women's sexuality

The main changes that affect women's sexuality are those that take place around the time of the menopause and afterwards. Menopausal symptoms such as hot flushes, night sweats, fatigue and mood swings may have a negative impact on a woman's sex drive. More specifically, the decline in oestrogen that happens at menopause can affect the urogenital tract itself, causing dryness and itchiness of the vagina and vulva. Women may find that they no longer produce so much vaginal lubrication during sexual arousal as they once did. This can be solved by using a lubricating gel or spending longer on foreplay.

▷ **Once the children have grown up and left home, partners are often able to revitalize the intimate side of their relationship.**

If you are suffering from menopausal problems that affect your enjoyment of sex, seek the help of a doctor or complementary therapist (a wide range of herbal and homeopathic remedies is available).

Although women's fertility declines around the time of the menopause, women who do not want to conceive should use contraception for at least a year after their last menstrual period. Barrier methods such as the condom or diaphragm are recommended and they do not interfere with hormone replacement therapy should you decide to take it. The natural, or "rhythm", method of contraception is not appropriate because ovulation becomes very erratic around the time of the menopause.

men's sexuality

Men may notice that their sex drive is lower in their 40s and 50s than it was when they were younger. They may also notice that that their erections are softer or smaller and at a less upright angle than they used to be. Ejaculation may be less intense and less forceful and the refractory period (the length of time before a man can have an erection after he has ejaculated) may increase.

Feelings of arousal are more likely to come from direct touch than, for example, visual cues such as the sight of a partner undressing. Sometimes these changes can have a positive effect on your sex life: because your sexual responses are slower and more focused on tactile stimulation you may be more sexually synchronized with your partner.

If you experience problems achieving or maintaining an erection, it is important to seek a medical opinion. Sometimes erectile problems are a warning sign of blocked arteries. Erection of the penis occurs because blood is actively pumped into the penile tissues – if your arteries are blocked then the blood is pumped less efficiently into the penis. Having said this, erectile problems can also result from stress or emotional problems. Try to reduce stress levels by giving your partner a soothing massage prior to sex and making the bedroom look as relaxing and welcoming as possible.

Health problems that affect sex

Some health problems become more common with age. These are the ones that can affect sexual function:
• Cardiovascular disease
• Diabetes
• Multiple sclerosis
• Alzheimer's disease
• Parkinson's disease

Sexual function may be affected by taking certain drugs including antidepressants, antipsychotics, beta-blockers and diuretic drugs. Occasionally, men who have prostate gland surgery may also experience changes in sexual function. You should consult your doctor about all of these issues.

▽ **Massage is a good way to rediscover the areas of your partner's body which enjoy attention the most**.

Sex tips for older people

Accept the changes that take place in your body and accommodate them. Spend longer on foreplay and make sex into a long, sensual encounter. Use massage oils and a lubricant if you need to. Introduce variety into your lovemaking by making love at unusual times in unusual places. Be experimental in whatever ways you like: use erotica, swap roles during sex, share sexual fantasies and read sex books together. The saying "use it or lose it" is particularly pertinent to sex as you get older. Staying sexually active keeps your sex organs functioning and maintains sexual desire. Remember that sexual activity does not have to mean intercourse; it can also mean extended foreplay, oral sex, masturbation (with or without a partner) or kissing and cuddling that makes you feel aroused.

Overcoming stress

Research shows that your stress levels can have a profound effect on your health. If you suffer from chronic stress you may exist in a permanent state of physiological arousal: your heart beat and blood pressure are constantly elevated and stress hormones such as adrenaline are circulating in your bloodstream. Chronic stress is implicated in a number of age-related health problems, the main one being cardiovascular disease.

what is stress?

Stress is a physiological survival mechanism. When you sense that you are under threat, the brain responds by sending a message to the adrenal glands on top of your kidneys, which, in turn, respond by releasing adrenaline. Adrenaline has effects on various body systems that, in combination, enable you to take action: to either run away from the source of the threat or to stay and fight it. This is known as the "fight or flight response".

Although this physiological response may have been useful in primitive times, when humans needed to literally fight or run away from sources of danger, it is less useful in modern society, where sources of threat are mainly psychological. For example, a contemporary source of stress

might be travelling to work on crowded public transport when you are already late for a meeting. Your brain registers stress but you will not be able to take advantage of the subsequent adrenaline rush because no physical action is necessary.

When instances of stress are occasional and short-lived, the body can cope (some degree of stress helps us to stay motivated and to meet our goals), but when they are frequent and long-lasting the body may be perpetually in a state of high alert. This is when your vulnerability to problems such as cardiovascular disease increases. For this reason, it is essential to find ways to overcome chronic stress as you get older.

dietary support

People often turn to "quick fixes" when they are under stress. They feel tired, irritable and lacking in energy and they often turn to chocolate, caffeine or alcohol for stress relief, or a quick energy burst. Unfortunately, these substances deplete the body of energy and make you feel worse.

The most important nutrients to include in the diet when you are under stress are the B vitamins, vitamin C, zinc, chromium and magnesium. Dietary therapists may recommend taking a multivitamin and

△ **Eating bananas rather than refined-sugar products can boost natural sugar levels, which helps to combat stress.**

mineral supplement that supplies these nutrients. It is also very important to avoid sugary foods when under stress because they stimulate the stress hormone cortisol. Instead, eat foods such as bananas, wholegrains, seeds, beans and lentils.

yoga, meditation and breathing

Learning relaxation techniques is a powerful antidote to stress. Yoga and meditation teach you how to still the mind

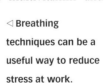

◁ **Breathing techniques can be a useful way to reduce stress at work.**

▷ **Relaxation techniques can help in the fight against stress-induced digestive disorders such as ulcers and indigestion.**

and focus on something simple such as the breath flowing in and out of your body. When you are stressed your breathing is usually fast and shallow. Making a conscious effort to relax your muscles and breathe deeply can help you to overcome stress. Yoga and meditation techniques are best learned from a trained therapist or teacher, but there are also plenty of books available.

One useful meditation technique is the humming bee practice. Sit in a comfortable position and close your eyes. Focus on the breath entering and leaving your nostrils. Say to yourself: "I am aware of breathing in. I am aware of breathing out". Use your fingers to close your ear flaps and imagine the sound of a humming bee inside your head. Breathe in and, as you breathe out, make the sound of a humming bee. Breathe in and repeat. Try to concentrate on the sound and on your breathing. Regular practice of this exercise should help to still your mind.

aromatherapy and massage

A range of complementary therapies can help to ease stress: acupuncture, reflexology, hypnotherapy, homeopathy and flower remedies. Aromatherapy and massage are very widely used in the treatment of stress and aromatherapists recommend the following essential oils: basil, bergamot, clary sage, camomile, geranium, hyssop, juniper, lavender, marjoram, thyme, cedar, neroli, rose and sandalwood. Massage can help to ease stress by relieving muscle tension and enhancing circulation.

Try a stress-relieving bath consisting of 2 drops each of camomile and marjoram, and 4 drops of juniper. Alternatively, try a drop each of camomile, juniper and marjoram dropped onto a tea bag and put in a large cup of hot water during times of stress.

personal stress-beaters

Everyone has their own ways of overcoming stress and it is important to cultivate methods that work for you. Some people unwind by talking to friends or a partner or by being sociable, others relax by spending time on their own. Exercise is a stress-beating technique that works for many people as it uses up adrenaline. The

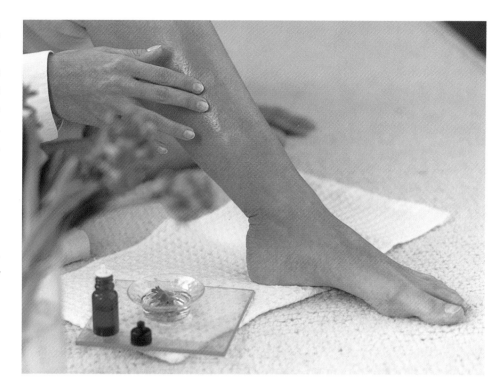

△ **Taking time to massage yourself with stress-relieving essential oils can be a good antidote to stress.**

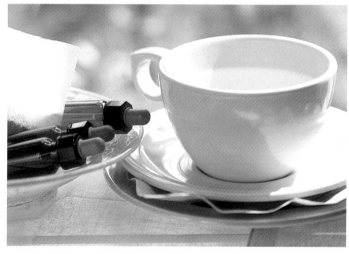

▷ **Herbal teas and Bach Flower Remedies are quick and effective cures for stress**.

endorphin rush that exercise brings can also provide a sense of well-being.

Sometimes a change of attitude can turn a stressful situation into a non-stressful one: ask yourself if a situation can be turned to your advantage in any way. Some people decide that, rather than trying to relieve the symptoms of stress, they will tackle the underlying cause. This may involve leaving a stressful job or ridding yourself of other responsibilities you can no longer manage.

Pet ownership can have a remarkable effect on stress levels. Pets act as morale boosters by offering unconditional loyalty. They can provide a valuable outlet for people who find it difficult to express their emotions – this in itself is cathartic.

▷ **By allowing us to care for them, pets can make us feel needed and appreciated.**

understanding depression

Many psychologists make a distinction between depressed mood and depression. Depressed mood describes the temporary sensation of "feeling down" that you have when something goes wrong in your life. Depression, on the other hand, is more intense and long-lasting. It can affect your behaviour, your relationships, your eating and sleeping patterns and your entire world view. The likelihood of depression may increase as you grow older. Elderly people, in particular, are more prone to suffering from depression.

recognizing the signs

Feelings of dejection, hopelessness and inadequacy are the most common signs of depression. But depression can manifest itself in a variety of ways and it is important to be aware of the signs, both in yourself and in others.

• Loss of interest in everyday activities
• Excessive sleeping or insomnia
• Fatigue and lack of energy
• Feelings of hopelessness and worthlessness
• Loss of sexual interest
• Apathy
• Excessive overeating or undereating
• Dejection, sadness and crying
• Problems with concentration and remembering things
• Difficulty making decisions
• Indifference to the world around you
• Suicidal thoughts and urges

what causes depression?

Depression can be triggered by a specific event. Life events that are associated with depression include divorce, separation, bereavement (particularly of a close family member), or being fired or made redundant. Sometimes depression has no specific or obvious cause. Depression that occurs in older people may result from a perceived loss of control in life. The prospect of growing older may in itself be depressing,

△ **Getting at least 15 minutes of bright sunlight and fresh air every day, preferably by taking a brisk walk in full daylight, can help to banish feelings of depression.**

especially given the fact that many societies tend to devalue aging and equate power and sexuality with youthfulness.

self-help for depression

If you feel depressed, try to make sure that you continue to eat and sleep properly. Avoid resorting to destructive props such as alcohol, cigarettes or drugs. Make sure that your diet is high in vitamin C, B vitamins, essential fatty acids and unrefined carbohydrates. Avoid refined, sugary foods.

If possible, stay active, exercise regularly (the endorphins released during exercise can help to combat depression) and seek the support of friends and family. Speak about how you are feeling and do not be afraid to express negative emotions such as fear, guilt, anger or sadness. Complementary therapies may help to combat depression. Herbalists

▷ **Taking time out to practise meditation may help you to relax and forget your worries.**

△ A sluggish digestive system can cause and increase feelings of depression, so ensure a high fibre intake is maintained.

◁ Vitamin C is essential in the fight against depression, yet it is depleted by stress.

recommend taking St. John's wort for depression, although long-term use of the herb may cause sensitivity to light. Aromatherapists say that essential oils such as basil, bergamot, clary sage, camomile, geranium, lavender, thyme, jasmine, neroli (orange blossom), rose, sandalwood and ylang ylang can help to lift mood, especially if used in combination with massage.

Understanding some of the cognitive processes that underpin depression can be helpful. The cognitive psychologist, Aaron Beck, says that depressed people often make "errors" in their thinking. If possible, try to challenge the following thought processes when they happen to you:

• Overgeneralization: the depressed person makes sweeping, negative generalizations. For example, "my whole life is pointless".

• Selective abstraction: the depressed person focuses on small negative details. For example, from a list of compliments, the depressed person remembers a chance remark that could be construed as negative.

• Magnification and minimization: the depressed person dramatizes the importance of negative events and downplays the importance of positive events. For example, a man who is not invited to a party sees himself as a social failure despite the fact that he has recently had an enjoyable meeting with some old friends.

• Personalization: the depressed person takes responsibility for things beyond his control. For example, "Today's train strike has happened because I need to get somewhere urgently".

• Arbitrary inference: the depressed person infers something without justification. For example, a woman infers from her husband's angry expression that she has done something wrong. If she had enquired further she would have discovered that her husband was angry about something unrelated to her.

△ Time spent making your surroundings more enjoyable can enhance your appreciation of life.

△ A warm, relaxing bath using uplifting aromatherapy oils can help against depression.

seeking professional help for depression

If you are suffering from depression you should consult your doctor. Treatment for depression consists of anti-depressant medication or psychotherapy, sometimes a combination of the two. There are different types of psychotherapy ranging from counselling to cognitive therapy to psychoanalysis. Discuss with your doctor which type meets your needs. If you are taking any complementary medicine, inform your doctor.

Thinking positively

Optimism, enthusiasm and a refusal to tolerate boredom are characteristics that are often associated with young people. There is no reason why this should be the case, however, and one of the best ways to remain psychologically young is to cultivate the art of positive thinking.

foster a sense of optimism

Life brings many experiences: some positive and some negative. As people get older they may fall into the trap of focusing on negative experiences and unwittingly cultivating a sense of pessimism about the future.

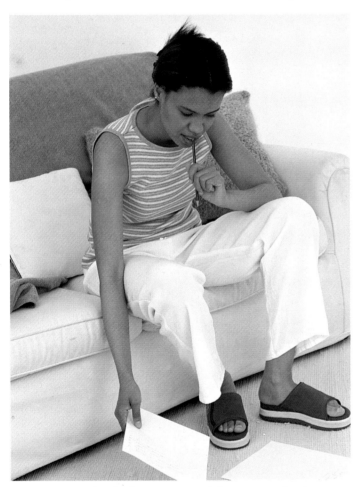

Pessimism can be further encouraged by media messages that value youth and denigrate aging.

Resolve to clear out your emotional baggage and foster a sense of optimism about the present and the future. Optimism has huge benefits for both psychological

and physical health – it can even boost your immunity to illness. Make a list of the life experiences that have affected you positively and negatively. Compare the positive list with the negative list. Ask yourself if anything from the negative list can be discarded or turned into a positive situation. Congratulate yourself on your achievements in life and concentrate on the future rather than the past.

Optimism is cultivated by keeping busy and active. Take up activities that make you feel good about yourself such as yoga, walking or swimming. Learn something

◁ By making a list of positive and negative aspects of our lives, we enable ourselves to see the areas needing attention.

▷ Planning a holiday can cheer you up by giving you something to look forward to.

completely new. Make sure that you are always working towards new goals and challenges. Set up a timetable in which to meet these goals. For example: "by the end of the year I will have converted one room of the house into a studio for painting, reading and music practice".

distance yourself from problems

If there are situations and problems in your life that you find inescapable, try to distance yourself from them. Take an overview: tell yourself that this is one episode in your life and it will not last indefinitely. If possible, try to see humour in difficult situations. Imagine that you are a stranger walking past the window of your own house. What would the stranger see? What would the stranger make of the events going on?

Ask yourself whether your current problems will still affect you in a year's time

or in five or ten years? If you can, let go of things that you cannot change and concentrate on the things that you can. Remember that, even if you cannot change a situation, you always have the option of changing the way that you think about it. Cultivate a sense of control.

Lock up your problems

When you are confronted with a negative situation or a problem, try the following visualization technique. Imagine that you have a small wooden box with a lock and key. Visualize the people or situations that are upsetting you and then open the box and carefully place them inside. Lock the box and put the key in your pocket. Place the box in a dark drawer and tell yourself that it stays there until you are ready to take it out and unlock it. When you are ready to deal with it, then do so. In the meantime, if the problem becomes greater, visualize taking the box out of the drawer, giving it a shake, and then replacing it.

have a mental clear-out

One negative stereotype of aging is that our beliefs become more rigid and inflexible as we get older. Challenge this assumption by discarding old beliefs and values. A belief that you have held for years may no longer be useful to you, it may be outdated or experience may have taught you new lessons. Question your beliefs about everything from gender roles to politics. Also question your beliefs about yourself. If you find yourself thinking you are incapable of doing something, ask yourself why.

Have a physical clear out as well as a mental and emotional one. If you make the symbolic gesture of throwing out clothes and other possessions that you have not used for years, this will reinforce your feelings of positivity and change.

enjoy the simple things

Think positively about small things in life as well as big things. Derive pleasure from everyday activities such as cooking meals, bathing and reading a book or newspaper. Immerse yourself in whatever you are doing. Take the time to look at your surroundings. If you always travel by public transport, try making the effort to walk once in a while.

Friendships are important in helping us to think positively. Friends provide support, companionship, humour and affection, as well as a valuable buffer against stress.

▷ Dogs have an unlimited capacity for enjoyment which can be infectious.

▽ Taking time to enjoy the company of a good friend can change a dull day into a good one.

The importance of sleep

Sleep is essential to your mental and physical well-being. If you do not have sufficient sleep, you are likely to become moody and bad-tempered. If your insomnia is chronic, you may be permanently tired, lacking in energy and depressed. Although sleeping patterns change as you grow older, getting a good night's sleep remains essential for the regular rejuvenation of the body.

why do we need sleep?

Sleep experts are not sure about the precise functions of sleep but it is thought that the body needs a period of rest every night to allow it to recuperate from the day and to repair cellular damage and maintain the immune system. Cells all over the body have the chance to regenerate and the brain consolidates what has happened during the day into long-term memory. People who are deprived of sleep may suffer from mood swings, irritability and psychoses.

sleep and aging

There is a popular misconception that people need less sleep as they grow older. In fact, your sleep requirements remain fairly constant throughout adulthood. Most people need approximately eight hours a night whether they are young or old. However, a variety of changes take place in sleeping patterns as people grow older and these changes conspire to make the overall duration of sleep shorter than before.

Sleep experts say that the "architecture" of sleep changes with age. Older people spend less time in deep sleep or "delta sleep" than younger people. Although they continue to spend the same amount of time in dream or "rapid eye movement" (REM) sleep as younger people.

People may find it more difficult to get to sleep as they grow older and this may be because they produce less of the chemicals that control the sleep/waking cycle. For

△ **If menopausal hot flushes keep you awake during the night, keep a fan, sponge and water beside your bed, so that you can easily cool yourself down.**

example, older people secrete less melatonin, a sleep-promoting substance produced by the pineal gland in the brain.

Other age-related changes to sleeping patterns include waking up more frequently and spending more time awake during the night. Generally, people adapt to these natural changes and do not find them debilitating.

problems with sleep

There are a number of specific problems that affect people's sleep as they grow older. For example, menopausal women may find their sleep is disrupted by hot flushes or night sweats. Typically, women wake up at intervals throughout the night feeling hot, feverish and drenched in sweat. They may need to change their bed clothes and bed linen, which adds to sleep disruption. In the long term this can lead to poor concentration, irritability, depression and reduced immune system efficiency. If your sleep is severely disrupted by night sweats, you should consult your doctor.

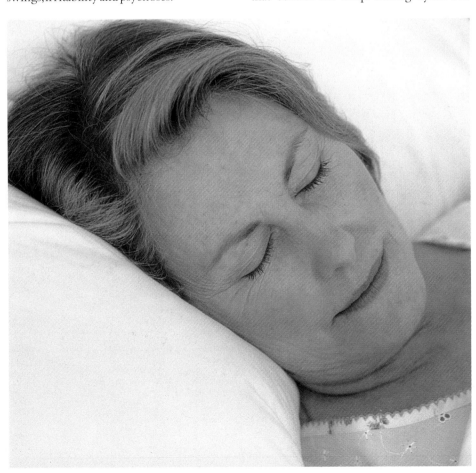

◁ **Skin cells regenerate at a much faster rate during sleep, so a good night's rest is important to a healthy body.**

△ **Making your bedroom welcoming and relaxing can help to induce sleep.**

Immediate self-help measures include keeping a bowl of water, a sponge, a hand-held fan and a towel by your bedside. Always wear night clothes made of natural fibres and keep a change of night clothes beside the bed.

Some age-related illnesses may interfere with sleep patterns. The aches and pains associated with arthritis can make it difficult to get to sleep and can disrupt sleep throughout the night. Digestive problems such as gastro-oesophageal reflux can abbreviate sleep. This is a disorder where

there is a backflow of stomach acid into the oesophagus. Sufferers may find that sleep problems can be resolved simply by raising their heads up off the bed.

Other age-related illnesses that can interfere with sleep patterns include cancer, osteoporosis, Parkinson's disease, bladder problems and cardiovascular disease. Some prescribed medications may also be responsible for disrupting your sleep. Diuretic drugs may cause you to get up frequently during the night to visit the bathroom.

Insomnia can sometimes have a psychological origin. If you are depressed, upset or anxious, for example, then sleep is

likely to be elusive. You should consult your doctor if you frequently suffer from chronic insomnia – it is important that the underlying cause is diagnosed and treated correctly.

On the other hand, a daytime nap can be a valuable way to relieve fatigue and sleepiness. If your night sleep is temporarily being disrupted and you are not usually an insomnia sufferer, a short nap during the day (before 3:00 pm if possible) can revive and refresh you, and give you the energy to keep going through the remainder of the day.

▽ **Try to take cat naps before 3:00 pm to avoid disturbing your ability to fall asleep at nightime.**

Daytime napping

Opinions are mixed about the value of napping during the day. If you are suffering from insomnia, it can exacerbate it. Also, rather than compensating for insomnia, you should try to discover and treat the underlying cause. On the other hand, by training our bodies to accept short periods of sleep when we need it we can avoid overstretching our systems during the day.

Quality sleep

coping with snoring

Snoring increases with age. It is not usually a sign of a serious problem, although it can disrupt the sleep of a partner. Snoring results when the airways are obstructed, usually because the muscles that keep them open are too lax or because there is a build up of fatty tissue around the airways. Anything that encourages muscle relaxation, from lying on your back to drinking alcohol, may make snoring worse. The noise of snoring comes from the air rattling over the relaxed tissues of the palate and throat.

Snoring is most common in middle-aged people who are overweight. There are several preventative measures:

• Lose weight.
• Avoid drinking alcohol or eating heavily before you go to bed.
• Sleep without a pillow.
• Quit smoking. Smoking is a major cause of airway congestion.
• Sleep on your side rather than on your back. You can force yourself to do this by sewing a tennis ball into the back of your nightclothes.

sleep apnea

Occasionally, snoring may be associated with a serious disorder known as sleep apnea which becomes more common in middle and later life. Sleep apnea occurs when the upper airway becomes blocked and prevents you from breathing. In severe cases, sleep apnea may result in high blood pressure and increase your risk of heart attack and stroke.

During the night the apnea sufferer stops breathing, levels of oxygen in the bloodstream fall rapidly and the sufferer wakes up briefly, gasps for breath and then falls asleep again. This happens over and over again throughout the night and often means that the sufferer feels extremely sleepy during the day. Sleep apnea may be accompanied by loud snoring and is most common in overweight or obese people. If sleep apnea is mild, it may be overcome by

△ **Practising relaxation exercises before going to bed may help you to overcome insomnia.**

◁ **A lavender sachet beside the bed, or a few drops of lavender oil on your pillow may enduce sleep.**

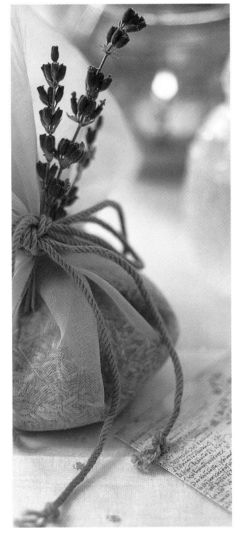

weight loss, lying on your side and avoiding smoking, alcohol and sedative medications. If it is severe, a doctor may recommend keeping the airways open with a special device or, sometimes, with surgery.

learning to relax

One of the best ways of enhancing sleep is learning an effective method of relaxation. Complementary therapies, such as aromatherapy, massage, acupuncture and flower remedies, can help you to relax and overcome insomnia. T'ai chi and yoga are also very useful. Or you can try the following creative visualization exercise.

Lie flat on your back with your arms by your sides, palms up, and your legs straight and hip-width apart. Breathe in and out deeply. Try to draw the breath down into your abdomen so that your lungs are taking in the maximum amount of oxygen to replenish your body. Close your eyes and focus your thoughts on a single item that

▷ **A warm aromatherapy bath before bedtime can relax muscles and emotions.**

▽ **Leave an aromatherapy burner alight whilst you prepare for bed to help your body and mind relax.**

you find relaxing, such as a cloud, a tree, a lake or the sea. Concentrate on the qualities – the texture, depth, colour and movement – of the image you have chosen. If any distracting thoughts come into your head, acknowledge them and then visualize them as leaves being gently blown away. Keep breathing deeply into your abdomen. When you are ready to finish your relaxation session, do so slowly. Let your thoughts return to the room you are in and gently move your toes and fingers. Roll onto one side and get up. Alternatively, you can do this exercise in bed before you go to sleep.

Enhancing sleep quality

Try to maximize your sleep quality by making your environment as comfortable as possible and by developing good sleeping habits.

- Make sure your bedroom is relaxing, warm and well aired.
- Burn lavender essential oil in an aromatherapy burner in your bedroom. Or put a handkerchief with a few drops of lavender oil under your pillow.
- Avoid eating a heavy meal immediately before going to bed.

△ **Some foods, such as turkey, avocado, cottage cheese, milk and bananas contain tryptophan which may assist healthy sleep.**

- Avoid caffeinated drinks or alcohol before you go to bed. Although alcohol can speed up the onset of sleep, it disrupts the pattern of sleep at a later stage in the night.
- Go to bed at roughly the same time every night (preferably earlier rather than later).
- Get up at roughly the same time every morning, even if you go to bed later than usual.
- If possible, use your bedroom for sleep only (rather than for work, watching television or talking on the telephone, for example). This way your brain will learn to associate the bedroom with sleep.
- Make sure your bed is comfortable and supports your spine. If you have a back problem, try sleeping on your side with your knees bent and a pillow between them.
- Cut out any sources of light that may keep you awake.
- Eliminate irritating noises. Fix dripping taps and noisy plumbing or radiators. Alternatively, buy some good quality ear plugs.
- Wear night clothes made from natural fibres.
- Have a warm bath and a milky drink before going to bed. Try the following essential oils in your bath: 2 drops each of camomile and rose with 4 drops each of juniper and marjoram, or 2 drops each of camomile and juniper and 4 drops of neroli.

△ **Listening to relaxing music before bedtime helps many people to switch from an active to a passive state of mind.**

- Eating foods that contain the amino acid tryptophan may help you to sleep. These include avocado, turkey, cottage cheese, milk and bananas.
- Do something relaxing and enjoyable, such as reading a book or listening to soothing music, before you go to bed.

Taking Care of Your Appearance

As you grow older the skin loses its natural elasticity and the hair becomes prone to greying and thinning – for many people these are the first visible signs of aging. There are some good techniques for preventing or accommodating changes in your appearance. It is worth remembering that if you are happy about the way you look this has an inspiring effect on your mood, making you feel more positive, confident and sociable.

Protecting the skin

△ **Add evening primrose oil or vitamin E to face cream to help rejuvinate mature skin.**

The skin is our largest organ and it serves as a protective barrier against bacteria and other invaders. As you age, your skin loses its elasticity, it gets thinner and it starts to wrinkle. In fact, the appearance of the skin is one of the main criterion that we use to judge a person's age. But, although the aging process results in skin wrinkling, it is only partly responsible: ultraviolet light from the sun also plays a large role.

how the skin ages

A protein called collagen is responsible for keeping the skin supple, elastic and youthful. When the skin is exposed to ultraviolet light from the sun, collagen fibres are attacked and destroyed. Although you lose collagen naturally with age, exposure to the sun greatly accelerates this process (so does cigarette smoking). Ultraviolet rays also damage the layer of skin where new cells are formed. The shape of the cells changes and they become smaller. This causes the skin to lose its thickness and become more translucent. Skin ages at a different rate on different areas of the body. Two of the first places that wrinkles appear are the hands and the face because both are constantly exposed to the elements. The skin on the neck, which is very mobile, is also prone to visible loosening and sagging with age.

Sebaceous glands, which secrete a lubricating substance onto the surface of the skin, become less active with age, resulting in dryness and flakiness.

common skin problems

Apart from wrinkling and sagging, there are some specific skin problems that are more likely to occur with age. These include broken veins and itchiness.

Broken veins become more visible as the skin ages and becomes translucent. As with age spots, broken veins do not require any special treatment. If broken veins are particularly unsightly, however, they can be removed using techniques such as electrocautery.

Itchiness of the skin may sometimes be associated with the menopause. A persistent sensation of tingling or itchiness around this time is known as formication. Some doctors may recommend hormone replacement therapy (HRT) to treat this irritating condition, as well as other menopausal symptoms.

taking care of your skin

The single most effective way to prevent premature skin aging is to protect your skin from the ultraviolet rays of the sun. This means avoiding exposure to intense sunlight whenever possible, covering your skin and wearing a sun hat on sunny days, and getting into the habit of always wearing a high protection sunscreen or sunblock.

Another way to protect your skin is to minimize free radical damage to body cells (free radicals are highly reactive substances produced during oxidation) from cigarette smoking and pollution. Avoid exposure to cigarette smoke (or quit smoking yourself) and environmental pollution, and eat foods that are rich in vitamins A, C, and E, betacarotene and selenium or zinc. These nutrients help to fight free radicals in the body; you can also take them in supplement form. Skin health can also be enhanced by making sure that you always have sufficient quality sleep.

Other dietary habits that will keep your skin youthful include the following:
- Limit your intake of tea, coffee, alcohol, sugar and saturated fat.
- Take an evening primrose oil supplement. This contains essential fatty acids that are needed by skin cell membranes.
- Drink plenty of pure water. Dehydration affects the skin and makes it dry.
- Increase the amount of fruit and vegetables in your diet, especially red, orange and yellow ones.

There are some "external" habits that you can adopt to preserve your skin. Try not to wash your skin too often and avoid harsh soaps that strip the skin of oil. Add oil to bath water and use good quality moisturizers (preferably containing sunscreen) on your body, hands and face. Moisturizers prevent the top layer of the skin from drying out but they cannot restore lost collagen.

△ **Drinking water not only hydrates the skin but also helps to flush away toxins.**

△ Applying the contents of a vitamin E capsule to your face once a week can help to soften aging skin.

beauty tips

Cosmetic products and procedures – and even cosmetic surgery – are frequently presented as a panacea for age-related problems. Unfortunately, they are often expensive and do not yield any long-term benefits. The alternative to shop-bought products are safe and simple techniques and practices evolved over hundreds of years from complementary therapies such as herbalism and aromatherapy.

stay moisturized

Even if moisturizers cannot restore lost skin tone, they can rehydrate the top layer of your skin, making it look firmer and healthier. To optimize absorption of moisturizer, apply it immediately after a bath when your skin is still warm and damp. Do not forget to moisturize your neck, an area which is much neglected and that is prone to sun damage.

Vitamin E is an important anti-aging vitamin for the skin which can be applied externally or ingested. Massage the contents of a vitamin E capsule into your face or, if you prefer to include vitamin E in the foods you eat, good sources include unrefined corn oil, sunflower seeds, sesame seeds, beans, wheatgerm and tuna.

Try the following recipe for calendula (marigold) cream. Mix 55g/2oz lanolin with 50ml/2fl oz wheatgerm oil. Add a handful of fresh or dried calendula flowers and heat for approximately two hours. Strain the liquid, add two capsules of vitam in E and leave to set in a jar. Use as an everyday moisturizer.

You can also use essential oils to lubricate your skin. Use 15ml/1tbsp of a base oil, such as evening primrose or sweet almond oil, and add 1 drop of an essential oil such as frankincense, geranium, lavender, neroli (orange blossom), or sandalwood. Massage gently into the skin taking care to avoid the eyes.

take herbal baths

You can improve the way you look and feel by taking a relaxing and therapeutic herbal bath. Turn out the lights and place some lit candles around the bath. Make sure that the water is the right temperature. There are a wide variety of commercial aromatherapy and herbal products that you can add to a bath or you can try making your own. To make a herbal tea bag, place the herbs in the centre of a coffee filter. Fold it and sew the open edges closed with a needle and cotton. Alternatively, place the herbs into a piece of muslin and tie the material with ribbon. Hang the bag onto the bath and let the hot water run through it. For a calming bath, use equal parts of camomile, hops and passion flower. For a stimulating bath, use equal parts of peppermint, eucalyptus and lavender.

Aromatherapists recommend that you add essential oils to your bath water to benefit from their therapeutic effects. For a calming bath use four drops of lavender, four drops of neroli and two drops of geranium For a stimulating bath use two drops of lemon, three drops of peppermint and three drops of rosemary.

△ Add different essential oils to your bath water to achieve calming or invigorating baths; Lavender and camomile are very relaxing.

While you are in the bath you can give your eyes a treat by covering them with cold, damp teabags, cucumber slices, or cotton wool.

have a massage

Having a regular massage is an excellent way to increase circulation, calm the nervous system, relieve muscle tension, promote sleep and improve posture, vitality and mood. These, in turn, have a knock on effect on your appearance. If you can, have an aromatherapy massage on a regular basis. Alternatively, give and receive a massage with a friend or partner

When you give a massage, you should always lubricate your hands with a base oil, such as almond, wheatgerm or olive, first. Avoid giving massage to people who suffer from skin problems or health problems such as osteoporosis.

A natural face pack

As your skin ages, you may find that commercial face packs strip your skin of oils, especially if they contain clay. To make a natural face pack that will help to moisturize and condition older skin, mash together half an avocado (or one raw egg yolk) with a small amount of honey. Apply to the face avoiding the eye area, and leave on for approximately 10 minutes. Use this face pack every week.

Hand and foot care

Hands are a good indication of the state of the body and many therapists use them as diagnostic tools when judging general health. Dry or brittle nails, for example, may reveal a lack of B vitamins, white flecks may indicate a lack of zinc, and weak nails could be caused by a calcium deficiency.

how the hands age

As you age, the skin on your hands tends to become dry and fragile, the nails may thicken and become ridged or they may get brittle and prone to breaking. Veins become more pronounced, age spots appear and the hand becomes thinner and less fleshy.

common hand problems

As you grow older it is common for age spots to appear on the backs of the hands. Age spots, sometimes known as liver spots, are due to melanin-producing cells clumping together with age. Melanin is a pigment produced by the skin that gives rise to the characteristic brown colour of a suntan. When melanin-producing cells clump together they produce distinctive brown spots or patches. Although age spots are not thought to be harmful, they can be

△ You should try to remember to moisturize your hands at least twice a day.

removed using laser or chemical treatment. Massaging the hands with saffron oil may also be helpful. Age spots may be worsened by cold weather and exposure to the ultraviolet rays of the sun, so always wear sunscreen on the hands in summer and gloves in winter.

Arthritis can cause problems such as pain, restricted movement and dexterity and even disfigurement in the hands as you grow older. Arthritis should receive medical diagnosis and treatment, but self-help measures include taking painkillers and applying alternate hot or cold compresses to the hands. Hand massage can also be helpful.

To give a massage, lubricate your hands with base oil mixed with a few drops of marjoram essential oil and gently sandwich one of the sufferer's hands in between both of yours. Gently stroke the length of the hand from the wrist to the fingertips. The warmth of your hands will ease the pain. Now gently rub and stroke the thumb.

looking after your hands

Moisturize your hands as often as possible, but at least once in the morning and evening, and after immersing your hands in water. Moisturizer is absorbed into the skin most quickly when it is warm, so apply it to warm hands or keep a bottle near to a source of heat.

Cleaning dishes in hot water that contains detergent can take its toll on your hands over many years. A good way to prevent skin damage is to cover your hands in handcream and put rubber gloves on before washing up. The warmth of the water will enhance the skin's absorption of the moisturizer.

Once a week, soak your fingertips in warm olive oil (or cider vinegar if you have weak nails) for 10 minutes. Then gently rub a teaspoon of salt into your hands. The abrasive action of the salt will remove dead skin cells. Now trim your nails using a pair of nail scissors, and file them into shape. Use an

△ Light nail polishes and shorter nails are more flattering for older hands.

emery board and sweep from the outer corner of the nail inwards. Push the cuticles back with an orange stick wrapped in cotton wool. Now buff your nails to smooth away ridges and give them a natural shine.

Always try to wear at least a clear nail polish to protect your nails against everyday wear and tear. If you are applying a coloured nail varnish, always use an undercoat first to prevent the pigment from sinking into the nails and causing staining. A top coat can double the length of time required between manicures by preventing chipping.

Skin aging on the hands

The backs of the hands are often the first place where skin starts to age. Try pinching the skin on the back of your hand for a few seconds and then release it. The rate at which it falls back into place varies according to age.

Under 30: 1 second

30–40 years: 1–2 seconds

40–50 years: 2–5 seconds

50–60 years: 10–15 seconds

△ Add a few drops of peppermint essential oil to baby oil and massage to relieve tired feet.

foot care

Years of wear and tear combined with badly fitting or poorly designed shoes can have an adverse effect on the feet as you grow older. You can also add to the burden by trimming the toenails badly or neglecting problems such as dry skin, corns and bunions. Good foot care is an important investment in your mobility – present and future.

common foot complaints

Corns and calluses are caused by friction between shoes and the bony areas of the foot. The bony parts of the foot become less padded with age, making corns and calluses

△ To nourish the skin add a handful of dried milk to a warm footbath and soak your feet for at least 15 minutes.

more likely. Prevention consists of wearing padded insoles, padding vulnerable areas of the feet and wearing well-fitting shoes. You can treat corns and calluses using over-the-counter medication.

Ingrown toenails occur when the toenail pierces the skin of the foot, and are most common on the big toes. This problem is usually caused by trimming the toenails in the wrong way. To prevent ingrown toenails, always cut the nail square across and level with the top of the toe. Never taper the sides of the nails or poke scissors or other implements underneath the nail. If you suspect that you have an ingrown toenail, visit a doctor or chiropodist (podiatrist).

Bunions are painful and severely retard mobility. They are caused by the overgrowth of bone tissue, and although the problem is often hereditary, it can be exacerbated by wearing ill-fitting shoes. A bunion is characterized by a swollen, tender big toe joint that protrudes from the foot. In mild cases, the bunion can be accommodated by wearing wide-fitting shoes or a protective pad on the toe joint. In severe cases, the foot can become misaligned and medical attention is necessary. Your doctor may recommend drug treatment or surgery.

Skin cracking around the heel becomes common with age. A self-help treatment is to soak your feet in warm water, then cover them with petroleum jelly, and put on a pair of cotton socks before going to bed. You can also alleviate dry skin by increasing the amount of essential fatty acids in your diet. Essential fatty acids are found in extra virgin olive oil, sunflower seeds and oily fish. You may also benefit from taking a vitamin E supplement or a tablespoon of linseed oil every day. If cracking is severe, dietary therapists may recommend taking 30mg of zinc twice a day over an eight-week period.

Even if you do not suffer from cracked skin, moisturize your feet after bathing. Skin on the foot is drier than elsewhere on the body, so try to use specially designed foot care products. If your feet sweat excessively, soak them in a bowl of warm water mixed with a handful of dried milk instead of applying moisturizer. Another useful remedy for dry, tired feet is a few drops of peppermint oil, added to some baby lotion and rubbed into the skin after bathing.

△ Regular use of a pumice stone after bathing can stop hard skin building up.

looking after your feet

Babies are born with fat, padded feet, but as you grow and your bones form, the feet become leaner and more defined. As you age the padding on the feet lessens still further and the feet become wider. Because your feet change throughout life, it is essential to have your feet measured periodically so that you can buy shoes that fit correctly. Choose socks that are the right size for your feet and whenever you have the chance, go barefoot. Another aspect of good foot care is a regular visit to a chiropodist (podiatrist).

The following tips can help to maintain the health of the feet and prevent problems.
• Give yourself a foot massage using essential oils mixed with a base oil.
• Avoid exposure to cold temperatures.
• Make sure that your socks do not impede circulation.
• Avoid sitting with one leg crossed over the other.
• Promote circulation by flexing and pointing your toes and circling your ankles, especially if you sit still for long periods of time.
• Sit with your feet raised if possible.
• Treat your feet to a warm foot bath and apply a special foot moisturizer afterwards.

Footcare for diabetics

The feet are particularly vulnerable to infection in people who suffer from diabetes (adult-onset diabetes becomes more common as you age). If you have diabetes, pay careful attention to foot care and consult your doctor about any foot problems, even minor ones such as corns and calluses. Avoid self-help treatment and visit a chiropodist regularly.

Healthy hair

As we age our hair tends to get thinner and turn grey. These tangible signs of aging are ones that many people try to prevent or conceal. As a result we spend much time and money on styling, colouring, treating and transplanting hair. Ultimately, many age-related hair changes are hard to prevent because they are genetically controlled. But this does not prevent us from having hair that is healthy and attractive.

△ **After shampooing, rinse your hair with warm water until the water runs clear and clean.**

△ **Having a fringe is flattering on older people as it can often soften their appearance as well as help to hide forehead lines.**

how the hair ages

On average we lose between 70 and 100 hairs per day. When we are young we replace these lost hairs with new ones but, as we grow older, hair loss speeds up and new growth slows down. Some hair follicles become sluggish and have long resting phases, other hair follicles appear to be completely deactivated. The result of these changes is fewer hairs and the overall appearance of thinning. Women may notice that their hair starts to thin out around the time of the menopause. However, if you suffer from sudden or severe hair loss, consult your doctor.

Men are prone to a particular type of hair thinning known as "male pattern baldness". This is distinct from age-related thinning and it is genetically controlled. Hair follicles that are affected by male pattern baldness start to produce a new type of hair known as a vellus hair. These are thin and delicate and they only grow to a short length. Because they are difficult to see, vellus hairs may give the impression of baldness. Eventually, true baldness occurs as the follicles die completely. Men can usually predict whether they will go bald simply by looking at older male members of their family. Although men may suffer from thinning

and baldness of head hair, they may find that nasal and eyebrow hair begins to grow more vigorously with age.

Hair that turns grey does so because of the loss of a pigment called melanin. As a hair shaft is produced, the hair follicle secretes melanin giving hair its characteristic colour. As pigment cells start to die – but some melanin is still produced – the hair has a grey colour. When the pigment cells die completely, the hair is white. Unpigmented hair has a characteristic coarse, wiry texture. Many people start to develop grey hairs in their 30s and 40s and hair becomes progressively more grey with age.

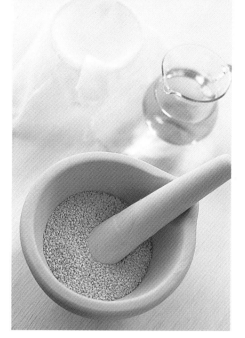

△ **Use as few chemicals as possible, instead opt for natural products such as sesame conditioner.**

looking after your hair

The key to having attractive and healthy hair as you get older is to wear it in a style that suits you and to keep it in optimum condition. This does not mean buying expensive hair products; in fact, the major determinants of hair health are regular exercise, a well-balanced diet and adequate sleep.

- Grey hair can be concealed with temporary or permanent colouring. Choose a shade that is lighter than your original colour. You may need to experiment with different products – the way in which your hair responds to colorants depends on how porous your hair shafts are.
- To condition dry, brittle hair, boil 3 tablespoons of ground sesame seeds in a little water for 10 minutes, strain through muslin and allow to cool. Massage the mixture into the hair and leave for 10 minutes before rinsing thoroughly.

▷ **Always gently comb conditioner through the hair to ensure it is evenly distributed and reaches as many hairs as possible.**

- Aromatherapists recommend the following tonic to revitalize hair: mix 10 drops of cedarwood essential oil, 10 drops of juniper essential oil and 15 drops of rosemary essential oil in 50ml/2fl oz of surgical spirit (alcohol). Massage a small amount of this mixture into damp hair and leave to dry naturally. Wash your hands afterwards.
- Dietary therapists recommend eliminating coffee, tea and sugar from the diet in order to promote hair health. Useful nutrients include essential fatty acids for dry or brittle hair, zinc for poor hair growth and a general multivitamin and mineral supplement for overall hair health.
- Avoid drying out your hair using hot hair dryers or styling tools, and try not to use bleach – it strips the hair of natural oils. Use an intensive conditioning treatment on your hair once a month.

Menopausal changes to hair

Oestrogen receptors are present in hair follicles and when oestrogen levels fall at the time of the menopause the growth and rest cycle of the hair is disrupted. Many women notice for the first time that their hair is thin, fine and difficult to style. This change is completely natural. Although you cannot reverse hormonally-related hair thinning (except with hormone replacement therapy) you can help to minimize hair loss by treating your hair gently. When you wash your hair, mix a mild shampoo with some water and then pour the mixture over your head. Leave it for a minute and then massage very gently and rinse off with warm water. Dab your hair rather than rubbing and comb with a wide-toothed comb. Leave your hair to dry naturally.

◁ **Herbal hair rinses use natural ingredients to leave your hair shining and well conditioned.**

▷ **Comb wet hair with a wide-toothed comb to gently free any tangles.**

Menopause

The menopause is the permanent cessation of the menstrual cycle, bringing to a close the period of life in which it was possible to bear children. It usually occurs between the ages of 45 and 50, although both early and late menopause are not unusual. While the prospect of the menopause may seem daunting, you should try to not to worry unduly. You can reduce the likelihood of suffering physical or psychological problems by adopting a positive attitude towards this new stage in your life.

The changing menstrual cycle

To understand what happens during menopause, it is important to know about the sequence of finely tuned hormonal events that takes place in the normal menstrual cycle.

the menstrual cycle

At the beginning of every menstrual cycle, a hormone is released from the brain called follicle-stimulating hormone (FSH). It stimulates the development of egg follicles in the ovary. As the follicles develop they produce the hormone oestrogen. One egg follicle eventually becomes dominant and releases an egg – a process known as ovulation – which travels down the fallopian tube. The follicle that produced the egg is left behind on the ovary where it starts to secrete the hormone progesterone.

As the egg travels down along the fallopian tube, the uterus, under hormonal direction, is preparing itself for a possible pregnancy. Oestrogen makes the uterine lining thicken and progesterone stimulates the growth of blood vessels so that the uterus is ready to receive a fertilized egg. If fertilization does not happen then the egg and uterine lining are simply shed from the body in a process known as menstruation.

In most healthy young women, the menstrual cycle takes place on a fairly regular basis – about every 28 days on

△ Irregular periods may be stabilized by adding 4 drops each of rose, camomile and melissa to a warm bath.

average. Several factors can change or disrupt the menstrual cycle, such as stress, illness, losing an excessive amount of weight or taking the contraceptive pill. The biggest changes, however, come with menopause.

changes to the cycle

As women grow older the brain releases follicle-stimulating hormone (FSH) in the way that it always has done, but the ovary does not respond in the usual way. With age there are less follicles left in the ovary to be stimulated, and the ones that remain may be of insufficient quality to make it to ovulation. This has several results: the brain increases the amount of FSH to "force" the ovary to respond, the remaining follicles

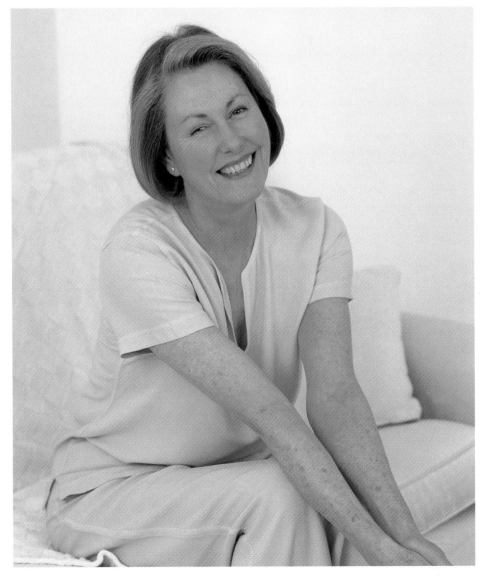

◁ The menopause usually occurs between the ages of 45 and 50, although both early and late menopause are not unsual.

△ **Regular exercise helps keep the body in balance by regulating body fluids and reducing fluid retention.**

produce less oestrogen than normal and, if ovulation does not happen, no progesterone is secreted.

These are the kinds of disruptions that take place in the menstrual cycle during the build up to the menopause. Ultimately, oestrogen levels go into permanent decline and ovulation becomes erratic and ceases, causing progesterone production and periods to stop as well.

the menopause timetable

Menopausal changes rarely happen suddenly. They usually take place over years. You may notice that your periods become more frequent and longer in duration. Or you may notice that your periods become infrequent with less blood loss than usual. Or you may alternate between both patterns. It is difficult to know what to expect. Some women skip periods for several months and then suddenly start menstruating again.

The word "menopause" refers to a single event rather than a series of ongoing changes: it is a woman's last ever menstrual period. This cannot be identified when it is happening – it can only be identified retrospectively. A more accurate word to describe the ongoing hormonal changes of midlife is the "perimenopause". Or some doctors use the word "climacteric". The postmenopause describes the years between the last period and the end of a woman's life.

- Premenopause: periods are still regular but symptoms may start to appear.
- Perimenopause: periods become unpredictable and symptoms may worsen.
- Postmenopause: periods stop permanently and, in time, the body adjusts to low hormone levels.

the age of menopause

Most women become menopausal in their 40s and 50s. The average age of menopause is about 51 years, although perimenopausal signs may be apparent before this age. Premature menopause takes place before the age of 35 and delayed menopause takes place after the age of 55.

It is likely that, as individuals, we are biologically programmed to reach menopause at a certain age. There is no link between the age of menopause and age of first menstruation or first pregnancy. Taking the contraceptive pill is not thought to influence the age of menopause. The age at which your mother was menopausal may affect the age of your menopause, but this is not conclusive. Smoking and low body weight, however, have been found to bring on the menopause earlier.

△ **Practising relaxation exercises can help to harmonize your body and alleviate symptoms of the menopause.**

▽ **The more positive an outlook you have on life, the fewer physical and psychological problems are likely to occur at the time of the menopause.**

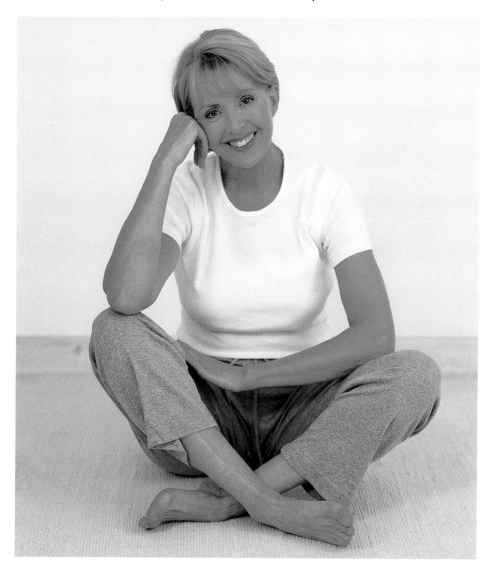

Symptoms of the menopause

Although some women experience very few problems at menopause, others begin to experience an array of symptoms that affect both the body and mind. One of the main reasons for this is the fact that oestrogen influences many different body functions. In fact, special receptor cells for oestrogen are present all over the body and in the brain.

why the menopause causes symptoms

Some experts have compared the symptoms of oestrogen decline to drug withdrawal: when supplies of oestrogen start to become erratic the body reacts negatively; if oestrogen levels are restored, the body gets its "fix" and returns to normal. Eventually, the body adapts to low oestrogen levels but this is something that may take years. Problems may also result from the fact that hormones released in the brain such as follicle stimulating hormone (FSH) can become unusually high.

Much research focuses on the importance of oestrogen but it is now thought that progesterone (or its absence) may also be important. After menopause, progesterone production stops completely whereas small amounts of oestrogen are still produced (fat cells produce oestrogen). This relative imbalance, coupled with progesterone deficiency, is thought to be a cause of troubling symptoms.

Warning signs

Menstrual upheavals are common around the time of the menopause but you should consult your doctor if you experience any of the following:

- Bleeding between periods
- Heavy bleeding with clots
- Bleeding after sex
- Bleeding following a year without periods

Common symptoms

Symptoms are many and varied as the hormone levels in the body fluctuate. Some of the most common symptoms are:

- Hot flushes and night sweats
- Palpitations
- Breast changes
- Mood swings
- Depression
- Poor memory
- Insomnia
- Tiredness
- Poor concentration
- Loss of sex drive
- Vaginal dryness
- Urinary problems
- Fluid retention
- Weight gain and shape change

▽ **Wearing cotton clothes, drinking iced water and using a battery-operated fan can help to ease the symptoms of hot flushes.**

hot flushes and night sweats

The most easily identifiable symptoms of the menopause are hot flushes and night sweats. Blood rushes to the face, neck and chest and you become hot, flushed and sweaty. Afterwards you may feel very cold. This can happen very frequently, sometimes several times an hour. When it happens at night, you may wake up drenched in sweat and feeling hot and feverish. Self-help measures:

- Find effective ways of cooling down. Carry a battery-operated fan or an insulated flask of iced water with you.
- Wear cotton or other natural fibres.
- Wear clothes that can be unbuttoned at the neck.
- Keep a record of when you have hot flushes and see if you can recognize a pattern. Are there any specific triggers?
- Avoid spicy food, caffeine and alcohol.
- Learn to relax and practise creative visualization techniques.

palpitations

Many women experience palpitations at the same time as they have a hot flush. However, they can also appear independently of hot flushes. The heart feels as though it is racing or beating irregularly and some women feel as though they are having a panic attack. Self-help measures:

• Take a break and sit or lie down.
• Close your eyes, inhale deeply through your nose and take the breath down into your abdomen.
• Tell yourself that the feeling is temporary and will soon pass.

△ **Aromatherapists recommend the use of clary sage against hot flushes and night sweats.**

△ **St John's Wort, recommended for lifting depression and stabilizing mood swings, can be taken as a tea, a tincture or a supplement.**

◁ **Keep a diary of menopausal symptoms – there may be a pattern to hot flushes and palpitations.**

▷ **Creating a relaxing atmosphere can help to ease palpitations, mood swings and depression.**

breast changes

The most common type of menopausal breast change is mastalgia. The breasts typically feel swollen, tender and painful to the touch. Self-help measures:

• Wear a good quality bra that supports your breasts. Wear a bra in bed if necessary.
• Cut down on the amount of saturated fat that you eat.

mood swings and depression

Fluctuating hormone levels may give rise to emotional problems such as irritability, crying fits, angry outbursts and anxiety. This is because oestrogen receptors in the parts of the brain that control mood are deprived of oestrogen. Disrupted sleep due to night sweats may give rise to mood swings. Feeling tired all the time will lessen your ability to cope. Self-help measures:

• Seek the support of your friends, family and partner. Explain to them how you are feeling.
• Talk to other menopausal women about their feelings or read the experiences of others. Join a self-help group.
• Learn relaxation and mood-lifting techniques that work for you.
• Try taking flower remedies or herbal remedies such as St. John's wort or kava kava (stop if you experience any side effects and if you are taking prescribed medications, consult your doctor).

More menopausal symptoms

poor memory

Forgetfulness often becomes a problem around the time of menopause. You may find yourself missing appointments or forgetting where you put things. The hippocampus, the part of the brain that is associated with memory, contains oestrogen receptors and may be less efficient at storing information when oestrogen levels start to decline. Self-help measures:

- Teach yourself to rely on diaries and lists. Keep exhaustive lists of everything that you need to remember.
- Keep a pen and a piece of paper by your bed and in your car.
- Highlight the most essential daily tasks that you must do. Tick them off at the end of the day.

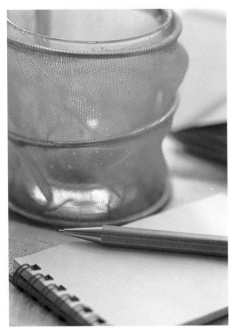

△ Keep a pen and paper beside the bed so that you can easily jot down important things that you remember during the night.

insomnia

The inability to fall asleep, waking frequently during the night and waking up too early are all classified as signs of insomnia. Suffering from insomnia may be a menopausal symptom in its own right or it may be caused by night sweats.

△ Massage relaxes the muscles and releases sleep-inducing chemicals in the brain.

tiredness

Feeling sleepy, apathetic or fatigued during the day can exacerbate other menopausal symptoms such as poor memory and concentration. Muscle fatigue is common during the menopause. Self-help measures:

- Accept your limitations: if you feel tired, try to rest rather than keep going.
- Avoid artificial stimulants such as coffee, chocolate and alcohol.
- Practise good sleeping habits (see Looking after the body).

poor concentration

Like poor memory, poor concentration is another cognitive deficit caused by declining or fluctuating levels of oestrogen in the body. Some people also find decision making more difficult than previously.

Self-help measures:

- Be lenient on yourself. Find out what your attention span is and work around it.
- Do not resign yourself to diminishing brain power. Stay mentally active.

loss of sex drive

Women notice that their sex drive decreases or even disappears around the time of menopause. This may happen spontaneously or it may be the result of an underlying problem such as vaginal dryness, breast pain, tiredness or depression. Self-help measures:

- Establish the underlying cause of the problem and, if possible, treat it.
- Remember that sex does not always have to be penetrative. Try being sexually intimate with a partner by cuddling or

giving each other a massage.

- Remember that postmenopausal women often experience renewed sexual interest.

vaginal dryness

Declining levels of oestrogen cause the urogenital tract to become thin and dry. The vaginal tissues shrink and less lubrication is produced than previously. This can make sex difficult and painful. Menopausal women may also be prone to vaginal soreness and minor infection.

Self-help measures:

- Insert a vitamin E capsule into the vagina nightly for a month and then whenever you need to.
- Use a natural lubricating gel, such as aloe vera or comfrey cream.
- Spend longer on foreplay during sex – the vagina may just be slower to lubricate than before.
- You should try and remain sexually active, as this will keep your reproductive system in good shape.

urinary problems

The urinary tract lies very close to the vagina and it also responds to declining oestrogen levels by becoming thin. The result of this may be discomfort on passing urine and frequent and urgent urination. Some women suffer from stress incontinence in which small amounts of urine escape from the body on laughing, coughing or picking up a heavy object.

Self-help measures:

- Drink 2 litres/3½ pints of water a day to keep the bladder flushed out.
- Practise Kegel exercises. These involve tensing the pelvic floor muscles (those used to stop urination) for a count of five. Repeat throughout the day.

fluid retention

A common feature of premenstrual syndrome, fluid retention, can become worse in the build-up to the menopause. You may feel bloated, swollen and heavy. If your weight fluctuates substantially, you should seek a professional diagnosis as you may have developed a food intolerance.

Self-help measures:

- Cut out salt, processed food and junk food.
- Eat foods that act as natural diuretics such as celery, parsley, chicory and dandelion.
- Avoid standing for long periods.
- Take plenty of exercise.

weight gain and shape change

Many women find that they put on weight during the menopause due to a lowered metabolism and a change in the way that fat is deposited in the body. Long-term low oestrogen levels also cause the body to change shape. The waist-to-hip ratio alters so that the waist thickens and comes out to meet the hips.

Self-help measures:

- Avoid faddish diets and calorie restriction at the time of the menopause. You need calcium and all the other nutrients that a normal diet supplies.
- Use exercise to control your weight and increase muscle tone.

△ **Natural diuretics such as celery, chicory, parsley and dandelion can help fight against fluid retention.**

▽ **Tightening and relaxing the muscles used to stop urination helps to prevent stress and incontinence.**

hormone replacement therapy

Hormone replacement therapy (HRT) is a type of medication that is designed to return a menopausal women's hormone levels back to her premenopausal levels. Doctors often prescribe HRT to treat debilitating menopausal symptoms such as hot flushes, insomnia and depression. HRT may also have a role in protecting women against the long-term health problems that are most frequently associated with the postmenopause such as osteoporosis and cardiovascular disease.

what is HRT?

HRT consists of the hormones oestrogen and progestogen (the synthetic form of progesterone). Oestrogen is widely considered to be the most important hormone in HRT; the role of progestogen is to induce a monthly bleed and to protect the uterus from cancer. Women who have had a hysterectomy may be prescribed oestrogen only.

The main advantage of HRT is that it may reverse many of the changes associated with menopause. This means that premenopausal body shape, skin and hair condition, sex drive and cardiovascular health can all be preserved and the classic menopausal symptoms are alleviated. The disadvantages are that women continue to bleed on a monthly basis (this is a withdrawal bleed rather than a proper period) and that HRT can cause side effects. HRT is also unsuitable for some women because of their medical history.

Some women feel that the menopause is medicalized in Western cultures and that taking medication during this time simply adds to the perception that the menopause is an illness or disease. This is a matter for debate: some people argue that women are suffering from a hormone deficiency disease that deserves medical treatment; others say that menopause is a natural rite of passage and the view that women are ill should not be encouraged.

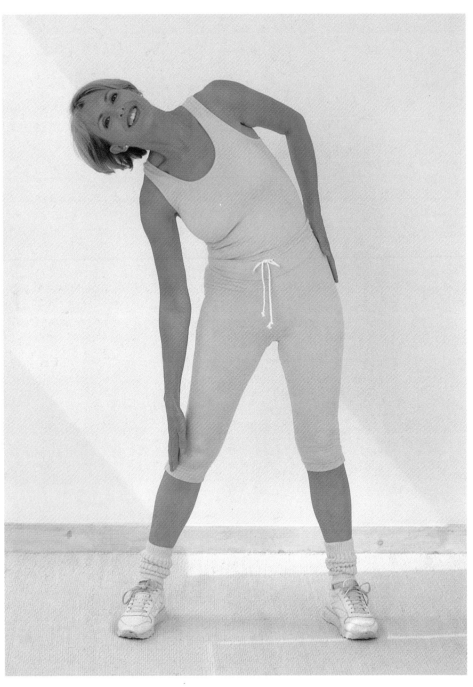

types of HRT

HRT is usually taken in pill form. The pills often come in calendar packs and you take one pill a day. All the pills usually contain oestrogen, whereas progestogen is only included in 10–14 pills in the latter half of the pill cycle.

Hormones can be absorbed through the skin and are available in the form of skin patches. The fact that hormones do not have to pass through the liver means

△ **Weight bearing exercise can help to prevent osteoporosis, as well as promote good circulation.**

that dosages are comparatively low and this may be an advantage for some women. The patches should be changed every three or four days.

HRT is also available in implant form. The implant is inserted under the skin in a minor surgical procedure carried out by your doctor. Although implants are convenient, in that you do not need to take pills or change patches, it is difficult to control the dosage. Localized symptoms of low oestrogen levels, such as vaginal dryness, may be treated with oestrogen cream or pessaries. However, this form of HRT does not ease other menopausal symptoms, such as hot flushes, and it does not have the long-term benefits of other types of HRT.

the possible side effects

It may take the body a while to adjust to the hormones in HRT and some women find that they are troubled by side effects even after several months of taking hormones. There are lots of different types, products, doses and regimes in hormonal medication and, ideally, HRT should be tailored to suit every woman's individual needs. If you are taking HRT and you experience side effects, consult your doctor about trying a different brand or type of HRT or changing the dose or regime. It may be necessary for you to take HRT for at least four months before your body adapts.

Your doctor may decide that HRT is not appropriate for you if you have any of the following:
• High blood pressure
• Endometriosis (in which the lining of the uterus grows outside the uterus)
• Benign breast disease, such as cysts
• Benign uterus disease, such as fibroids
• A history of thrombosis
• Migraine
• Ovarian or uterine cancer
• Pancreatic disease
• Liver disease
• Recent cardiovascular disease
• Breast cancer or a family history of breast cancer.

Research shows that taking oestrogen and progestogen may be associated with an increased risk of breast cancer. This does not rule out taking HRT altogether but the risks and benefits for each woman need to be assessed carefully by a doctor.

▷ **You should discuss any menopausal symptoms with your doctor to make sure that you receive the advice and treatment that you require during the menopause.**

Side effects of HRT

Some women may find that they suffer from side effects while taking HRT. These side effects may include:
• Headaches
• Nausea
• Impaired eyesight
• Breathlessness
• Premenstrual syndrome
• Heavy or irregular bleeding
• Breast tenderness
• Skin problems such as acne and itchiness
• Weight gain
• An increased or decreased sexual drive
• Muscular pains and backache

▷ **Some women find HRT patches more beneficial than tablets. Since the hormone does not have to travel through the liver, side effects are reduced.**

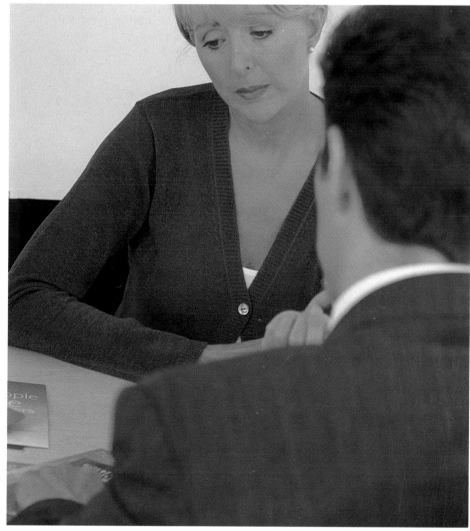

Natural alternatives to HRT

More and more women are turning to complementary therapies to help them through the menopausal years. A range of therapies offer gentle but effective ways to overcome symptoms and increase overall well-being. Although many therapies can be practised safely in the home, it can be helpful to seek the guidance of a therapist, at least in the first instance.

herbalism

There are many herbal treatments for menopausal symptoms and the best advice is to visit a medical herbalist who will tailor treatments to your individual needs. Herbal remedies come in a variety of forms including infusions, decoctions and tinctures – these can be made with fresh or dried herbs. There are also many commercial herbal supplements in the form of pills or capsules that are available in health food shops or some pharmacies.

Herbs that contain oestrogen-like substances – known as phyto-oestrogens – may compensate for declining oestrogen levels at menopause and ease many menopausal symptoms. Such herbs include panax ginseng, black cohosh, dong quai, alfalfa, liquorice and red clover. Remedies that are recommended for specific menopausal symptoms are as follows:

• Hot flushes and night sweats: agnus castus, sage, yarrow, motherwort

• Poor memory or concentration: ginkgo biloba
• Depression: St John's wort
• Anxiety: vervain
• Breast pain and pre-menstrual syndrome: evening primrose oil
• Insomnia: valerian, passionflower

Stop taking herbs if you experience any side effects. Consult your doctor before taking herbs if you suffer from high blood pressure or cardiovascular disease.

aromatherapy

The essential oils that are therapeutic at the menopause include sage, camomile, geranium, rose, jasmine, neroli, ylang ylang, bergamot and sandalwood. You can use these essential oils in the bath, in a massage (mixed with a base oil), you can burn them in an aromatherapy burner or you can put a few drops on a tissue or a pillow. Sage essential oil is thought to be good for hot flushes and ylang ylang is recommended for reviving the libido.

flower remedies

There is a wide choice of flower remedies available and you do not need to consult an expert before taking them. There is a range of flower remedies to suit various emotions and you can combine remedies to achieve the mixture that is right for your specific emotional symptoms.

homeopathy

A homeopath can assess your symptoms and choose the most suitable remedy and potency for you. Health food shops and some pharmacies also sell a standard range of homeopathic remedies. The remedies that are most frequently recommended for menopausal symptoms are as follows:

• Hot flushes: Lachesis, Sepia, Belladonna
• Breast pain: Bryonia
• Mood swings and irritability: Lachesis, Sepia, Pulsatilla
• Insomnia: Pulsatilla
• Premenstrual syndrome: Bryonia, Pulsatilla
• Vaginal dryness: Sepia, Natrum muriaticum

traditional Chinese medicine

Practitioners of Chinese medicine aim to restore the flow of energy, or Qi, through the body using acupuncture, acupressure and Chinese herbalism. Both herbs and acupuncture may be recommended for hot flushes. Always consult a registered doctor of Chinese medicine.

massage

Receiving massage can have a relaxing and therapeutic effect on both the mind and the body. If possible, visit a massage therapist and explain your symptoms. Regular massage can help to relieve insomnia, anxiety, depression and muscle and joint pain.

△ Sprinkle alfalfa shoots onto salads for a tasty and nutritious source of phyto-oestrogens.

△ The storage methods for herbs can vary greatly so always read the instructions carefully.

△ Essential oils, such as sandalwood, clary sage, or camomile, can have an uplifting effect.

yoga

A core benefit of yoga during the menopause is that it teaches you relaxation techniques that you can use at any time in your day-to-day life. The practice of breathing techniques (pranayama) can still the mind and relieve stress and anxiety. Meditation can also be of great benefit. The physical postures of yoga (asanas) can help to maintain flexibility and strength in the joints and muscles and bring balance to the body and mind. If possible, join a class and learn yoga from an experienced teacher.

△ This yoga position, known as the Child's pose, is an excellent relaxer for the body and mind.

dietary therapy

Research suggests that Asian women do not suffer as badly as Western women from menopausal problems and this is believed to be due to their soya-based diet, rich in phyto-oestrogens and calcium. It is worth experimenting by drinking two glasses of soya milk per day for a period of a month to see if you experience a lessening of symptoms. Other foodstuffs rich in phyto-oestrogens include oats, barley, wild rice, brown rice, wholewheat, celery (which is also useful against fluid retention), sprouts and green beans. Recommended supplements during menopause include evening primrose oil, vitamin C with bioflavonoids, vitamin E, and a general multivitamin and mineral supplement.

It is advisable to avoid the following in your diet around the time of the menopause:
• Caffeine
• Hot spicy foods
• Alcohol
• High sugar consumption
• High salt consumption
• High animal fat consumption
• Bran-based foods that may strip the body of nutrients such as calcium.

"Natural HRT" cake (7 day supply)

The following recipe for a natural HRT cake contains ingredients that are rich in phyto-oestrogens and vitamin E. It is low in fat and high in fibre and may help to alleviate symptoms of the menopause.

115g/4oz soya flour
115g/4oz wholewheat flour
115g/4oz porridge oats
5cm/2in chopped stem ginger
2.5ml/$\frac{1}{2}$ tsp ground ginger
2.5ml/$\frac{1}{2}$ tsp nutmeg
2.5ml/$\frac{1}{2}$ tsp cinnamon
200g/7oz raisins
115g/4oz linseeds
50g/2oz sunflower seeds
50g/2oz sesame seeds
50g/2oz sliced almonds
15ml/1tbsp malt extract
150 ml/$\frac{1}{4}$ pint soya milk

Sift the flour and add all the dry ingredients. Mix well before slowly adding the milk and malt extract. Cover and leave to soak for an hour. Spoon mixture into a cake tin lined with waxed paper and bake for up to 75 minutes on 190°C/370°F/gas 5. Allow to cool and eat one slice per day.

△ Store your HRT cake in an airtight container, and eat within seven days.

△ You should always wash fresh fruit and vegetables thoroughly before eating in order to rinse off any traces of pesticides.

Essential nutrient guide for the menopause

Take plenty of the following:
• Phyto-oestrogens: replace your usual milk and flour with soya milk and flour.
• Selenium-rich foods: wheatgerm, wheatbran, tuna, tomatoes and onions.
• Vitamin E-rich foods: sunflower oil, sun-dried tomatoes, seeds, almonds, unsalted peanuts, leafy green vegetables and eggs.
• Calcium-rich foods: tofu, cheese, leafy green vegetables, root vegetables, nuts and salmon.
• Magnesium-rich foods: brown rice, nuts, wholegrains and legumes.
• Potassium-rich foods: avocados, leafy green vegetables, bananas, nuts and potatoes.
• Zinc-rich foods: meat, mushrooms, eggs, wholegrains, nuts and seeds.
• Foods rich in vitamin B-complex: wholegrains, brown rice, milk, cereals, leafy green vegetables, fish, meat, eggs, avocados, seeds and yogurt.
• Vitamin D-rich foods: oily fish such as sardines, mackerel and tuna (vitamin D can also be obtained from exposure to bright sunlight).
• Water, juices and herbal teas to keep the body sufficiently hydrated.

Health checks

You should start to have regular health checks in middle age. Some, such as blood pressure tests, may be practised routinely by your doctor as you get older. Others, such as bone density scans, are specialized tests that may be performed if you are thought to be at particular risk of disease.

self checks

As you approach the menopause, keeping a diary of your periods and any physical and emotional symptoms you experience enables you to look for patterns and develop coping strategies. This information is also useful to your doctor. You should also perform a breast self-examination once a month and weigh yourself on a weekly basis to check that you are not gaining weight. If you are, you can take steps to lose it quickly.

blood cholesterol tests

Testing the blood for cholesterol is one way to assess your vulnerability to cardiovascular disease. If your blood cholesterol is too high, you can try to reduce it by making dietary changes. Blood cholesterol checks can be carried out by your doctor or it is possible to buy home-test kits.

blood pressure checks

Checking your blood pressure is a routine test that most doctors will carry out at regular intervals as you grow older. If your blood pressure is too high, you can try to reduce it through dietary changes, or your doctor may prescribe medication.

bone density scans

Postmenopausal women become more vulnerable to osteoporosis as they get older. Although it is not a routine health check, the best way to gain a picture of bone health is a specialized type of x-ray, known as a bone density scan. If you have already been diagnosed with osteoporosis, doctors may recommend bone density scans to assess the efficacy of any treatment you are having.

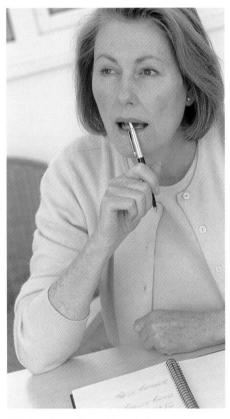

△ **By keeping a diary of health changes you may be able to give your doctor valuable information should their help be required.**

cervical smear tests

Cancer of the cervix affects younger women more than older women but, nevertheless, the cervical smear test remains an important diagnostic tool. It can show up precancerous changes in the cervix in women of all ages and action can be taken to prevent the cancer developing. You should have a cervical smear test every two or three years; more frequently if you have a history of genital warts.

If any abnormalities are detected during a cervical smear test, a doctor may perform a colposcopy. This is a technique that permits close-up inspection of the cervix at a microscopic level.

electrocardiograms

An electrocardiogram (ECG) is a specialized test that may be performed if your doctor suspects heart problems.

Electrodes applied to your body transmit electrical signals to a monitor. The signals appear as a trace on the monitor screen and provide detailed information about the contractions of the heart muscle.

eye tests

Because you become more susceptible to eye problems as you get older, it is important for you to visit an ophthalmologist annually. Eyesight problems can have serious repercussions with age and, when combined with weak bones, can increase the chances of falls and fractures.

hormone level tests

Testing the blood for the presence of elevated hormone levels can provide valuable information about the stage you are at in the menopause. For example, when the aging ovary fails to respond to follicle-stimulating hormone (FSH) the brain responds by releasing higher-than-usual amounts of FSH into the bloodstream. Hormone level tests are most likely to be performed by a gynaecologist.

mammography

The cure rate for breast cancer depends on the stage at which it is detected and whether or not it has spread. Mammography makes the early detection of breast cancer possible by providing an x-ray-type image that shows up changes in breast tissue. Mammograms are recommended every two years from the age of 45 (earlier if you have a family history of breast cancer).

other tests

There are other tests that your doctor may perform based on your individual medical history and current health. Both adult-onset diabetes and ovarian cancer, for example, can be detected by a blood test. You should try to keep abreast of the health tests that are available and ask your doctor about them.

△ **By performing breast examinations once a month, at the same point of the menstrual cycle, you will be able to detect any changes in the tissue at an early stage.**

breast self-examination

It is important that you examine your breasts regularly, once a month at the end of your cycle if you are still menstruating, and at any time if you have ceased menstruation. Standing in front of a mirror, look for any changes in shape or texture of the breast tissue or around the nipples. Do this first with your arms by your sides and then with your hands raised behind you head.

Lie on your back with your shoulders slightly raised. With the fingers of your right hand gently examine your left breast in widening circles from the nipple outwards. Then, using your left hand, repeat the examination on your right breast. Finally, raise each arm behind your head in turn and check the armpits.

Consult your doctor if you notice any unusual lumps, dimples, nipple discharge, or the inversion of a previously normal nipple.

Complementary health

Practitioners of complementary health use a variety of diagnostic tools and techniques to assess health and detect illness. Some are the same as those used by conventional medical practitioners, others may be less familiar. For example, naturopaths use x-rays and blood tests in the diagnostic process. Practitioners of Chinese medicine are more likely to look at the colour of your skin, the colour and coating of your tongue and feel the rhythm and strength of the pulses at the wrists.

▽ **Weighing yourself once a week, at the same time of day, not only checks against weight gain, but also detects weight loss which can be an early sign of some illnesses.**

Herbs for health

Most people are familiar with herbs that are commonly used in cooking, such as basil, bay, chives, mint, oregano, parsley, sage and thyme. But taking into account the broader definition of the term "herb", one can include plants such as aloe vera, spices such as ginger, flowers such as marigolds and roses, and fruits such as lemons and rose-hips.

As well as adding aroma and delicious flavour to food, culinary herbs have some nutritional value, often containing appreciable amounts of vitamins, minerals and trace elements. Adding herbs to your food on a daily basis actively promotes good health. Many herbs have excellent digestive qualities, helping the body to process and eliminate oily, fatty or gas-producing foods. But adding a generous sprinkling of fresh or dried herbs to your food is not the only way to benefit from these versatile plants.

herbal medicine

Many herbs have a therapeutic and medicinal value and can be taken in a variety of forms to prevent and cure illness and to promote health. Taken internally they can be made into herbal teas, decoctions, tinctures and inhalations. Externally they can be applied as compresses, poultices, ointments, creams or infused oils. Herbs add

▽ Pot marigolds, dried in the summer when they are plentiful, can be made into healing salves and ointments.

△ A tea infuser, available from health or cookware stores, is a useful gadget for making a single cup of tea from dried herbs.

their aroma to bath water for a therapeutic soak and essential oils distilled from the flowers can be used for a massage.

harvesting herbs

The best time to harvest the arial parts of herbs is after their flower buds have formed but before they are in full bloom. Roots should be dug up in the autumn, cleaned and chopped into small pieces. Never pick herbs without being able to correctly identify them, or pick so many that you reduce next year's growth.

Spread the herbs out to dry in an airy position out of direct sunlight – an airing cupboard is an ideal place. Leafy bunches can be tied into little bundles and hung up. Spread flower heads on tissue or newspaper and dry them flat. It can take a week for them to dry. The volatile oils in herbs start to deteriorate quickly once the herbs are put in the light. Store dried herbs in separate, airtight containers away from the light and they will keep for up to six months.

herbal teas

Herbal infusions make wonderfully refreshing drinks and can be drunk as caffeine-free alternatives to ordinary tea and coffee. Herbal teas can be taken to help ward

△ The antiseptic and antibacterial properties of thyme make it a first-choice tea for sore throats, colds and chest infections.

off colds and flu, to aid digestion, promote sleep, to relieve headaches, anxiety and stress, even to promote energy.

To make a herbal infusion, allow 30ml/ 2 tbsp fresh or 15ml/1 tbsp dried herb to each 600ml/1 pint/2½ cups water. For a single cup (250ml/8fl oz), use two small sprigs of fresh or 5ml/1 tsp dried herb. If you are using fresh herbs, wash them first, especially if they have been picked from the wild. Put the herbs into a warmed pot. Pour on boiling water. Replace the lid to prevent vapour dissipation. Leave to brew for three or four minutes, then strain the tea into a cup for a refreshing drink.

Drink a cupful of the appropriate tea no more than three times a day, and for sleep disturbances, drink a cup before going to bed. Teas can be stored for up to 24 hours in the refrigerator. Herb teas can be sweetened with honey to taste, but never add milk.

Caution

Herbs are powerful and can be harmful if taken in excess. Do not make teas stronger or drink them more frequently than recommended. Seek medical advice before taking herbal remedies when pregnant.

Herbal tea remedies

herb	treatment	herb	treatment

Teas for coughs and colds

Horehound
Marrubium vulgare

Make with the fresh or dried herb. Sweeten to taste with honey and add a dash of lemon juice. Take it for a chesty cold.

Purple Sage and Thyme
Salvia officinalis and *Thymus vulgaris*

Use in equal quantities in a tea to ease a sore throat. For a more powerful effect, add 1.5ml/¼ tsp cayenne pepper, which has antibacterial properties.

Peppermint, Elderflower, Chamomile and Lavender *Mentha x piperita, Sambucus nigra, Chamaemelum nobile* and *Lavandula officinalis*

At the onset of a cold, use 2.5ml/½ tsp of each of the first three, with a pinch of lavender, per cupful of water. Add a sprinkling of ground ginger, 5ml/1 tsp honey and a slice of lemon.

Hyssop
Hyssopus officinalis

For a cough, use the fresh or dried leaf, or the leaf and flowers. Hyssop is quite bitter, so sweeten this tea with honey and a little freshly squeezed orange juice, which adds valuable vitamin C.

Thyme *Thymus vulgaris*

Its antiseptic properties are good for chest infections. use 5ml/1 tsp dried thyme, or 10ml/2 tsp fresh, per cup. It has a warming effect and can also be used for digestive problems and stomach chills.

Teas for digestive troubles

Chamomile
Chamaemelum nobile

For digestive upsets, brew tea from the dried flowers. For a change, substitute half the chamomile for dried peppermint.

Peppermint and Lemon Balm *Mentha x piperita* and *Melissa officinalis*

Use fresh herbs in equal quantities for a pleasantly flavoured digestive tea to drink after a meal.

Fennel Seed
Foeniculum vulgare

For flatulence and indigestion. Crush the seeds and simmer in an enamel saucepan for 10 minutes before straining. This is also a traditional slimming aid and can help relieve hunger pangs. Caraway seeds can be prepared in the same way.

▷ **Limeflowers and elderflowers have a gentle soporific action as a night-time drink. Sweeten with honey to taste.**

Teas as tonics

Stinging Nettles
Urtica Dioica

A tonic tea to cleanse the system. It may also help alleviate rheumatism and arthritic pains. Chop up a small handful of young, fresh nettle leaves and infuse in 600ml/1 pint/2½ cups boiling water before straining.

Spearmint *Mentha spicata*

The tea has a zingy, uplifting taste. Use 15ml/1 tbsp chopped, fresh leaves per cup and sweeten to taste.

Basil *Ocimum basilicum* var. *album*

Calming to the nervous system, it also helps relieve nausea. Add 3–4 fresh leaves per cup.

Teas for disturbed sleep

Chamomile
Chamaemelum nobile

One of the best bedtime drinks for those who have difficulty getting to sleep. It is calming to the nervous system, as well as a digestive. Make it with 5ml/1 tsp dried chamomile to a cup and try adding a pinch of lavender for extra relaxation.

Limeflower and elderflower
Citrus aurantiifolia and *Sambucus nigra*

A pleasant bedtime tea. Add a dash of grated nutmeg and sweeten with honey.

Valerian
Valeriana officinalis

Use the dried and shredded root for a tea to calm the nerves. Using 10ml/1 tsp to a cup of water, simmer gently for 20 minutes in an enamel pan with a lid. Let it cool, then strain, re-heat and drink.

Teas for headaches, anxiety and depression

Rosemary
Rosmarinus officinalis

One of the more pleasant tasting teas when made with the fresh herb. Put one or two small sprigs per person into a teapot or cup and add boiling water. Rosemary is invigorating and refreshing. It clears the head and helps to ease headaches. Add a few betony leaves to relieve nervous tension if you prefer.

Lemon Balm
Melissa Officinalis

For tea, always use the freshly gathered herb. It has a long tradition as an anti-depressant.

St John's Wort
Hypericum perforatum

Use fresh or dried leaves and flowers. It helps to relieve nervous tension, anxiety and depression.

Herbal beauty treatments

Many of the old herbals included advice on using herbs for beauty, and making prefumed preparations was part of the apothecary's art. The following recipes are not soley cosmetic but are directed towards therapeutic beauty treatments and will promote general health through an enhanced sense of well-being.

dry skin moisturizer

Moisturizing cream prevents dryness of the skin, keeps wrinkles at bay and protects your skin from the weather. If you prefer, substitute dried elderflowers for the pot marigolds. Splash a little tonic on to your face first to feel refreshed.

120ml / 4fl oz / ½ cup water
20ml / 4 tsp fresh or 10ml / 2 tsp dried marigold petals
30ml / 2 tbsp emulsifying ointment
5ml / 1 tsp beeswax
30ml / 2 tbsp almond oil
2.5 ml / ½ tsp borax

Boil the water and pour over the dried marigold petals in a jar. Leave to stand for 30 minutes then strain.

Put the emulsifying ointment, beeswax and almond oil into one bowl and the elderflower infusion and borax into

▽ **Pot marigolds are recognized for their ability to soothe all manner of skin irritations.**

△ **There can be few pleasanter ways of dealing with stress and anxiety than sitting back and breathing in the therapeutic fragrance of essential oils.**

another. Set both over hot water and stir until the oils melt and the borax dissolves.

Remove from the heat and pour the elderflower mixture into the oils. Stir gently until incorporated. Leave to cool, stirring at intervals. Pour into a jar before it sets.

Rose petal toner

Infusions of flowers and herbs make excellent skin toners. Apply with cotton wool (cotton balls) after removing a face mask or make-up, or use at any time to freshen the skin. These toners must be kept chilled and used up within a few days as they soon deteriorate. Any fragrant roses are

Caution

Be aware that herbs are a potent source of medicine, containing essential oils and potentially therapeutic properties that can be harmful if misused, or used in larger quantities than specified. Pregnant women should avoid all kinds of herbal remedies unless under professional supervision.

△ **Dark red roses are the best for colour. The toner on the left is made from fragrant 'Ena Harkness' roses.**

suitable for this recipe, as long as they have not been sprayed with pesticide. Pink or red ones are best.

40g / 1½ oz fresh rose petals
600ml / 1 pint / 2½ cups boiling water
15ml / 1 tbsp cider vinegar

▽ **A steam treatment relaxes and softens the skin. Make it with an infusion of dried herbs, or simply float fresh herbs in boiling water.**

Put the rose petals in a bowl, pour over the boiling water and add the vinegar. Cover and leave to stand for 2 hours, then strain into a clean bottle.

chamomile steam facial

An occasional facial steam treatment deep cleans the skin. The heat relaxes the pores and boosts blood circulation. With the addition of herbs, the stimulating and cleansing action of the steam is increased. Always close the pores afterwards by dabbing with a cooled skin toner appropriate to your skin type or by using a face mask. Steam facials should be avoided altogether by those with a tendency to thread veins.

40g / 1½ oz fresh or 15g / ½ oz dried chamomile flowers
600ml / 1 pint / 2 ½ cups boiling water

Make a strong infusion of the fresh or dried flowers in boiling water. Leave to stand for 30 minutes, then strain. Re-heat the infusion, pour into a bowl and, keeping your

▽ **A herbal foot bath restores and revitalizes the whole body.**

face about 30cm/12in above the steam, cover both head and basin with a towel for about 30 seconds. Take a short break and then repeat two or three times.

herbal foot bath

There is nothing like a fragrant foot bath for refreshing tired feet. At the same time, it revitalizes the whole being, its warmth relaxes the body and the scent of the herbs calms the mind. Foot baths are also comforting if you have a cold.

50g / 2 oz mixed fresh herbs: peppermint, yarrow, pine needles, chamomile flowers, rosemary, houseleek
1 litre / 1¾ pints / 4 cups boiling water
15ml / 1 tbsp borax
15ml / 1 tbsp Epsom salts

Roughly chop the herbs, put them in a large bowl and pour in the boiling water. Leave to stand for 1 hour. Strain, and add to a basin containing about 1.75 litres/3 pints/7½ cups hot water – the final temperature of the foot bath should be comfortably warm. Stir in the borax and Epsom salts. Immerse the feet and soak for 15–20 minutes.

Variation

For a quick alternative foot bath, instead of making an infusion float fresh chamomile flowers and leaves in hot water. You could also use mint, marjoram, marigolds or rose petals. Or, for extra fragrance, try adding a few drops of an essential oil such as lavender to the water.

glossary

agni fire, transformative force that drives metabolic processes such as digestion.

akhrot walnut.

ama a toxin that can be formed by both physical and non-physical causes, such as indigestible food or painful experiences.

amla/amala/amalaki the Indian gooseberry (*Emblica officinalis*).

analgesic reduces sensitivity to pain.

anaphrodisiac diminishes sexual drive.

antiallergic reduces sensitivity to various substances.

anticoagulant agent which stops blood from clotting.

antidiabetic prevents the development of diabetes.

antifungal prevents the development of fungus.

antilactogenic prevents or slows down the secretion of milk in nursing mothers.

antimigraine reduces or prevents migraines.

antiparasitic prevents the development of parasites.

antipruritic prevents itching.

antipyretic counteracts inflammation or fever.

antisclerotic anti-aging; prevents hardening of tissues.

antiseptic prevents the development of bacteria.

antispasmodic prevents muscle spasm, convulsion.

antitussive relieves or prevents coughing.

antiviral prevents the development of viruses.

arjun/arjuna extract from the bark of the arjun tree (*Terminalia arjuna*).

aromatology the study of essential oils for health, including intensive and internal use.

astringent causes contraction of living tissue.

badam almond.

baingan aubergine, eggplant or brinjal.

balsamic fragrant substance that softens phlegm.

besan chickpea or gram flour.

bhasmas medicines traditionally made from precious stones.

bibhitaki extract from the fruit of the beleric myrobalan tree (*Terminalia belerica*).

bindi decorative mark worn on the forehead.

brahmi oil infused with the Indian herb gotu kola (*Centella asiatica*).

capillary dilator dilates the capillaries, aids circulation.

cardiotonic has a tonic effect on the heart.

carminative relieves flatulence (wind).

chemotype visually identical plants with significantly different chemical components and properties, e.g. *Thymus vulgaris* phenol and alcohol chemotypes.

choleretic stimulages bile production in the liver.

cicatrizant healing; promotes scar tissue

dalchini cinnamon.

depurative purifying or cleansing.

dhania coriander or cilantro.

diaphoretic see sudorific.

dinacharya the Ayurvedic daily routine.

diuretic promotes the secretion of urine.

diya traditional ghee-burning lamp with a cotton wick.

emmenagogic induces or regularizes menstruation.

febrifuge reduces temperature, antipyretic.

fixed oil non-volatile vegetable oil.

gram flour chickpea flour or besan.

gulab rose petals.

gunas sattva, rajas and tamas, the three inner qualities of all things.

haritaki extract from the fruit of the Indian gall nut (*Terminalia chebula*).

hatha yoga the physical exercises that form a part of yoga.

hypertensor increases blood pressure in hypotensive person.

hypotensor reduces blood pressure in hypertensive person.

kapha dosha representing earth and water.

karma the result of our actions in this and previous lives.

kesar saffron.

kokum a sour fruit native to the west coast of southern India, usually available dried.

lactogen promotes the secretion of milk.

litholytic breaks down sand or small kidney or urinary stones.

lypolytic breaks down fat.

maceration the extraction of components from plants by steeping in fixed oil.

mahabhutas the five "great elements": earth, water, fire, air and ether (space).

manjishtha/manjista extract from the root of Indian madder (*Rubia cordifolia*).

margosa see neem.

marma point place where two kinds of bodily tissue or two different energies meet; prana may become blocked at these points.

mehendi the art of painting the hands and feet with henna.

methi fenugreek.

mucolytic breaks down mucus and catarrh.

multani mitti/mati fuller's earth.

neem Indian tree (*Azadirachta indica*), also known as margosa; all parts are used therapeutically.

neurotonic stimulates and tones the nervous system.

oestrogenic stimulates the action of the female hormone, oestrogen.

ojas the substance that holds body, mind and spiritual levels together.

panchakarma detoxifying procedure that may include enemas and nasal washes.

phlebotonic improves or stimulates lymph circulation; lymph tonic.

pitta the dosha representing fire and water.

prakruti the constitution at birth, with all the doshas present in the right balance.

purvakarma preparatory treatments before panchakarma, including steam baths and herbal oil massages.

rasayana treatments aimed at rejuvenation or regeneration.

rubefacient increases local blood circulation causing redness of the skin.

shatavari extract from the tuber of wild asparagus (*Asparagus recemosus*).

shikakai Indian soap nut; the ground pods of *Acacia concinna*, used to treat the hair.

shodhana the full detoxifying process, including purvakarma and panchakarma.

sindoor vermilion powder applied to a woman's hair parting during her wedding.

stomachic stimulates secretory activity in the stomach.

styptic arrests haemorrhage by means of astringent quality; haemostatic.

sudorific induces or increases perspiration.

swedana sweat therapy.

tadrak ginger.

tamas/the tamasic state the lowest state of mind: greedy, selfish, violent and dull.

triphala blend of three herbs, amla, haritaki and bibhitaki, to balance the doshas.

tulsi/tulasi holy basil (*Ocimum sanctum*).

ubtan a powder used for skin cleansing.

vasodilator causes blood vessels to increase in lumen (the hollow inside of the blood vessel)

vata the dosha representing space and air.

vikruti a person's current state, in which health and feelings are affected by the changing balance of the three doshas.

vulnerary promotes the healing of wounds.

yoga literally "union", a set of spiritual and mind–body practices, including the physical exercises called hatha yoga.

Useful addresses

United Kingdom

Aromatherapy associations
Aromatherapy Organizations Council
(AOC), P. O. Box 19834, London SE25 6WF
Tel: 020 8251 7912

International Society of Professional
Aromatherapists (ISPA)
ISPA House, 82 Ashby Road, Hinckley
Leics LE10 1SN Tel: 01455 647 987

International Federation of Aromatherapists
(IFA)
Stamford House, 2–4 Chiswick High Street,
London W4 1TH Tel: 020 8742 2605

Aromatherapy products
Shirley Price Aromatherapy Limited
Essentia House, Upper Bond Street
Hinckley, Leics LE10 1RS Tel: 01455 615 466

Specialized short courses in aromatherapy
Penny Price
Sketchley Manor, Burbage, Leics LE10 2LQ
Fax: 01455 617 972

Aromatic medicine and aromatology
Dr Robert Stephen
4 Woodland Road, Hinckley
Leics LE10 1JG Fax: 01455 611 829

Ayurvedic remedies and treatments
The Ayurvedic Shop, 299 King Street, London
W6 9NH Tel: (020) 8563 0303

Neem products
Bioforce (UK) Ltd, Brewster Place, Irvine
Ayrshire KA11 5DD www.neemco.co.uk

British Wheel of Yoga
25 Jermyn Street, Sleaford, Lincs NG34 7RU
Tel: (01529) 306 851 www.bwy.org.uk

Ayurvedic facelift
Savita Patel, 151 Drummond Street, London
NW1 2PB Tel: (020) 7388 9795
e-mail: savita@facelift.fsnet.co.uk

Transcendental Meditation
Freepost, London SW1P 4YY, Tel: (08705) 143
733 www.t-m.org.uk
e-mail: mail@tm-london.org.uk

Ayurvedic therapies and beauty treatments
Pinka Yusupoff, 95 Kenbrook House, Leighton
Road, London NW5 2QW Tel: (020) 7284
4883. e-mail: pinkayusupoff@aol.com

United States

Aromatherapy associations
National Association for Holistic
Aromatherapy
2000 2nd Avenue, Suite 206
Seattle, WA 98121 Tel: (888)-ASK-NAHA

Aromatherapy products
Adriaflor
188 Lancaster Road, Walnut Creek
CA 94595 Tel: (925) 935-3601

All Aroma
1324 Sinloa Drive, Glendale
CA 91207 Tel: (077) 81-AROMA

Aromatherapy Outlet
666 West 84th Steet, Hialeah
FL 33014 Tel: (35) 828-7655

American Yoga Association
P. O. Box 1998, Sarasota, FL 34276
Tel: (941) 927 4977
www.americanyogaassociation.org

Aromatherapy teaching
Aroma Studio
4 Taylor Road, Warwick, NY 10990

Nordbloom Swedish Healthcare Center
178 Mill Creek Road, Livingstone
Montana 59047, Tel: 406 333 4216

The Australasian College of Herbal Studies
P. O. Box 57, Lake Oswego, Oregon 97034
Tel: 503 635 6652

Ayurvedic treatments, products and training
Ganesha Institute for Ayurveda and
Vedic Studies
4898 El Camino Real, suite 203, Los Altos, CA
94022 Tel: (650) 961 8316
e-mail: info@healingmission.com

Australia

Aromatherapy products
Nature's Energies
P.O. Box 112, Upper Ferntree Gully
Victoria 3156. Tel: (03) 9779-4369

International Yoga Teachers Association
P.O. Box 31, Thornleigh, New South Wales
2120
Tel: (02) 9484 9848 e-mail: info@iyta.org.au

Ayurvedic consultations, products and training
OmVeda Beauty and Health Centre
P. O. Box 248, Rozelle, New South Wales 2039
Tel: (02) 9810 1830 www.omveda.com.au

France

Ayurvedic products and training
Vedicare, 7 Impasse St Pierre, 75020 Paris
Tel: 33 (0) 1 44 93 91 26 www.vedicare.net

India

*Ayurvedic treatments after personal consultations,
products, online courses*
Jiva Ayurvedic Research Institute
1144 Sector 19, Faridabad 121002, Haryana
www.ayurvedic.org

Northern Ireland

Aromatherapy products
Angela Hills, 32 Russell Park
Belfast BT5 7QW

Republic of Ireland

Aromatherapy products
Chritine Courtney, Oban Aromatherapy
53 Beech Grove, Lucan, County Dublin

Norway

Aromatherapy products
Margareth Thomte, Nedreslottsgate 25
0157 Oslo, Tel: 22 170017

index